Nursing from the Inside-Out:

Living and Nursing from the Highest Point of Your Consciousness

(Transform Yourself and Impact Your Nursing Practice Through the Art of Self-Care)

Rachel Y. Hill, BS, ARNP, FNP-BC
Certified Hypnotherapist
Certified Reiki Master Teacher
Certified Karuna Reiki Master Teacher
Certified Kundalini Yoga Instructor
Certified Circle of Life Coach
Certified Jin Shin Jyutsu Practitioner
Healing Touch Student–Apprentice
Chakra Balance Therapist
Clinical Herbalist Student
Kansas City, Kansas

JONES AND BARTLETT PUBLISHERS
Sudbury, Massachusetts
BOSTON   TORONTO   LONDON   SINGAPORE

World Headquarters

Jones and Bartlett Publishers
40 Tall Pine Drive
Sudbury, MA 01776
978-443-5000
info@jbpub.com
www.jbpub.com

Jones and Bartlett Publishers
Canada
6339 Ormindale Way
Mississauga, Ontario L5V 1J2
Canada

Jones and Bartlett Publishers
International
Barb House, Barb Mews
London W6 7PA
United Kingdom

Jones and Bartlett's books and products are available through most bookstores and online booksellers. To contact Jones and Bartlett Publishers directly, call 800-832-0034, fax 978-443-8000, or visit our website, www.jbpub.com.

Substantial discounts on bulk quantities of Jones and Bartlett's publications are available to corporations, professional associations, and other qualified organizations. For details and specific discount information, contact the special sales department at Jones and Bartlett via the above contact information or send an email to specialsales@jbpub.com.

The authors, editors, and publisher have made every effort to provide accurate information. However, they are not responsible for errors, omissions, or for any outcomes related to the use of the contents of this book and take no responsibility for the use of the products and procedures described. Treatments and side effects described in this book may not be applicable to all people; likewise, some people may require a dose or experience a side effect that is not described herein. Drugs and medical devices are discussed that may have limited availability controlled by the Food and Drug Administration (FDA) for use only in a research study or clinical trial. Research, clinical practice, and government regulations often change the accepted standard in this field. When consideration is being given to use of any drug in the clinical setting, the healthcare provider or reader is responsible for determining FDA status of the drug, reading the package insert, reviewing prescribing information for the most up-to-date recommendations on dose, precautions, and contraindications, and determining the appropriate usage for the product. This is especially important in the case of drugs that are new or seldom used.

Production Credits

Publisher: Kevin Sullivan
Acquisitions Editor: Emily Ekle
Associate Editor: Patricia Donnelly
Editorial Assistant: Rachel Shuster
Production Editor: Amanda Clerkin
Marketing Manager: Rebecca Wasley

V.P., Manufacturing and Inventory Control: Therese Connell
Composition: DSCS/Absolute Service, Inc.
Cover Designer: Kristin E. Parker
Cover Image: © Sarah Nicholl/Dreamstime.com
Printing and Binding: Malloy, Inc.
Cover Printing: Malloy, Inc.

Library of Congress Cataloging-in-Publication Data

Hill, Rachel Y.
   Nursing from the inside-out : living and nursing from the highest point of your consciousness / Rachel Y. Hill.
      p. ; cm.
   Includes bibliographical references and index.
   ISBN-13: 978-0-7637-6996-3 (alk. paper)
   ISBN-10: 0-7637-6996-7 (alk. paper)
1. Nurses—Health. 2. Self-care, Health. 3. Alternative medicine. I. Title.
   [DNLM: 1. Burnout, Professional—prevention & control. 2. Nurses—psychology.
      3. Complementary Therapies. 4. Self-Care—methods. WM 172 H647n 2011]
   RT67.H55 2011
   610.73—dc22

                                                                                 2009033404

6048

Printed in the United States of America
14 13 12 11 10   10 9 8 7 6 5 4 3 2 1

In memory of three very special women of great courage and inspiration:
Mary Burmeister, Charlie McGuire, and Janet Mentgen

Contents

Acknowledgments

I give thanks to God for all things. I am thankful to be able to share the sacred spaces of many nurses. Special thanks go to Jones and Bartlett Publishers for allowing me to bring a dream to reality. I would like to thank my children for their graceful adjustments to having a nurse for a mother. I am grateful to my family and friends for their love and support. Thank you, Marcus, for being my companion and my confidant and for keeping me focused during my many adventures. Thank you, Brad, Ced, and Cindy, for tending to our flock. Brad, you have been a vital part of my career success and I thank you for your support and friendship. Thank you, Eric, for the home-cooked meals and funny text messages. I thank my favorite nursing organizations, the American Holistic Nurses Association and the American Nurses Association, for their presence in the nursing community. I am grateful to the following people for their contributions to my formal and holistic education and to my life experience: Ariella Mirkin, Amrita Burdick, Dr. Linda Johnson, Kahla Wheeler, Linda Gentry, Jay Peters, Mary Oberg, Darryl Olive, Sat Inder, Karta Purkh, Rebecca McLean, Dr. Linda Bark, Jody Hueschen, Dr. Terry Martin, and the faculties at University of Tulsa, MidAmerica Nazarene University, the Research College of Nursing, the Healing Touch Program, Healing Touch International, and the American Institute of Holistic Theology.

Foreword

You know how flight attendants always instruct airline passengers on how to use the oxygen masks in an emergency? "Place the mask over your head first before you help someone you are caring for put his on." That just seems like common sense, and sitting there in our seats, we never question it. But this is not how we nurses usually operate. Our focus is on the OTHER, to our own detriment. We go around putting the oxygen on our patients first, without giving much thought to our own oxygen levels. We don't heed the flight attendant's message. We burn out, and many of us leave nursing or count the days until we retire.

For many of us, the idea of taking care of others comes not only from the nursing tradition, but also from our own upbringing and the role of being a woman. The two together deeply reinforce the message that taking care of ourselves means we are selfish and uncaring. How do we change this multigenerational message that has sunk deep into our cells and often directs our way of being and doing in both our professional and personal lives? This is not an easy task. It is like reprogramming ourselves at a very profound level. And, it has reverberations. The OTHER may not like it, even though in the long run, ignoring our own needs really doesn't work. We can become resentful and angry. Care coming from such emotions doesn't really feel good to either the giver or the recipient.

When (notice I don't say "if," because I honestly believe this will be a major contribution to health care in our country) 2.3 million nurses start taking care of themselves, it will be earthshaking and groundbreaking. Taking care of ourselves has enormous repercussions not only for us as nurses, with a ripple effect on our families and our clients, but also for our planet. How we care for our planet is mirrored in the way we care for our mother Earth. I am quite serious when I describe this issue of self-care as revolutionary.

Enter Rachel Hill and her book, *Nursing from the Inside Out*. This is exactly what we need: leadership in helping us make this shift from the OTHER to OURSELVES. She offers to be our guide and teacher on an extraordinary journey to a new land. And what we need to remember is that this is not about either the other or us. It is about both the other and us. We both get oxygen. This is really simply about who gets it first. We can give even more from a full cup than from an empty cup.

In the early 1970s, I taught a course in holistic nursing, and I remember one nurse in particular who took my class. Her goal was to have 15 minutes a day for herself, which was quite a feat since she worked full time in OB and had a husband and five children. It was an 8-week course, and each week she would put together a plan for getting that time to herself, and each week she would say that something had come up and she didn't get her time. She would have a busy day at work, or something would happen to one of her children and she needed to care for him or her. Finally, in the sixth week, she found a solution that worked for the rest of the course. After work, she drove to the park and sat on a bench under a tree, and took her 15 minutes. She said it made all the difference in the world to her, and she felt like it was the beginning of a new way for her to start meeting her needs.

Rachel helps us with that first step. . .that new way of being that allows us all to have that life-giving oxygen. She gives us just what we need to feel comfortable in what might be for some readers a strange land, full of new ideas and ways to care for ourselves. For those of us who are already on the self-care path, she offers support for what we are doing and ways to learn more. In each chapter, she discusses different self-care practices and provides a history of how each practice got started. Understanding the context and how each came into being provides a platform that allows me to be more comfortable with them. She explains concepts, myths, and facts along with practices and exercises. By the end of each chapter, I feel like I am standing on a strong foundation and know what to do—an amazing experience.

The whole book is written in a way that is so inviting. Because she is an excellent storyteller, I am pulled into each chapter by her "tell it like it is" approach. She is authentic and transparent, and I feel like I can trust her. I am able to see her doubts, struggles, and triumphs, so I feel like I have a partner on this path of self-care because I can identify with all of those steps she shares.

Her warmth and openness are matched by her skill in weaving together worldviews that some have a hard time combining. She can quote scripture on one page and move into an Eastern practice on the next. This ability to present East and West, North and South in an easy-to-read, respectful, and user-friendly manner stands out to me as a demonstration of her years of practice and own meaningful and multifaceted inner work.

This is exactly what we need in nursing. We want to take this message to heart for the sake of everyone. Thank you, Rachel Hill, for your pioneering and innovative work in the field of self-care. I am sure that anyone who reads this book will finish it feeling inspired, supported, and informed, and ready to take new actions on his or her self-care path.

Linda Bark, PhD, RN, MCC
Alameda, California

Preface

As far back as I can remember, I have known that I had a book percolating inside me. I would always walk around family gatherings boasting about my plans to impress the adults. "I am going to write a book when I grow up," I would say. They would always respond by asking, "What are you going to write about, Baby Rachel?" (Baby Rachel was my childhood nickname and is no longer permitted for public use). Feeling put on the spot, I would be embarrassed because I had not actually worked out the details or thought that far into the future regarding what I would actually write about. I would simply try to put them off by telling them, "It's a secret!" I knew eventually I would have to figure things out and make good on a confirmed topic for my great literary work!

About 20 years later, I finally came up with some content for a book: nursing bloopers! Well, I didn't actually come up with the content. My nursing experiences gave it to me! If you have the time, I could tell you stories for days. I have enough experience to create cartoons, comic strips, soap operas, and mystery novels—you name it! For instance, there was the time my tennis shoe stuck to the floor while I was carrying a 24-hour urine sample to the lab. The "pee and me" came tumbling down. Luckily it was the night shift, and no one was in the hallway when I took off streaking (faster than lightning) down to the employee showers! Let's just say the security staff got a good laugh and some very incriminating footage out of it.

Another time, I was looking for the milk-and-molasses enema that had been ordered for my patient. The Dietary Department had sent it up, but I couldn't find it. Eventually I learned that they had sent it up on the patient's lunch tray, without telling me. She drank her milk and dipped her rolls in the molasses for lunch. When she ran out of her bread, she decided to drink the rest of her syrup (I will never understand why). To make matters worse, she was a diabetic. I had to write up my very first incident report. So how is that for crazy content?

I really and truly could go on sharing more stories, because they are so memorable. I'm sure a lot of my experiences are very similar to some you have experienced and could share yourself. (If there is a nurse in this world who has slipped on a 24-hour urine sample, I would love to meet you.) However, the most important story I will probably ever share is about the day I decided to leave nursing. When look back at myself on that day, I am reminded of a little child who packs a backpack with a peanut butter and jelly sandwich, an apple, and a couple of toys, preparing to run away from home. Of course, the child only gets as far as her parents' backyard. I ran away. I had in my mind that I was going to do anything but nursing. I didn't get very far at all. In my efforts to find other meaningful careers, the "pink Cadillac" never panned out and my newly found career seemed to be missing a vital component. That missing piece was patient care.

At that point in my life, I had grown so tired of politics, unequal workloads, backbiting, misunderstandings, incorrect paychecks, large patient loads, ungrateful patients, unrealistic expectations, not enough resources, unfair holiday scheduling, and. . .you get the picture. In the thick of the madness, I had to sprinkle family time over all my chaos. Imagine how that worked out. Neglected self, neglected kids, and building resentment. In all my frustrations, an ever so tiny, still voice spoke to me. What that little voice actually said was, "Look beyond your profession and examine what's inside you." This voice was trying to tell me that I should look beyond nursing while I am looking at the problems with nursing. After I got over the realization that I could be creating my own burnout and dissatisfaction, and that I might be playing the "victim," I knew what I needed to do. I needed to change. This was a difficult pill to swallow. My choices, behaviors, and thoughts had more to do with my dissatisfaction with my job than they did with the job issues themselves.

What did I need to do? Simply put, I needed to stop blaming nursing for my disharmony, and learn to create peace and harmony in my life. I know I am not alone in being disgruntled with nursing. I have total empathy for anyone who takes on the challenges of our profession. I do think some of that emotion might be misdirected. My heart is touched to share this special message with you: There is a solution for every challenge. There are many real issues we face in nursing—the statistics regarding burnout and staff retention speak for themselves. Once I stopped blaming nursing for my personal and professional challenges, I began to seek ways to find inner peace. Once I started seeking ways to find inner peace, I became equipped to make different choices. Once I started making different choices, my life began to look like a beautiful and consistent place to be. The world became beautiful and consistent when I started treating myself like a rock star/princess/diva and honoring the inner voice that speaks to me. That, my friends, has been the most incredible journey yet. "I'm a soul having a human experience" is a common phrase I hear from many who describe this learning life we have on Earth.

My intention is not to infer that everyone who reads this book is standing on the threshold of burnout. But even if you've got it all together, there's a good chance that you might know someone who is or has been chronically frustrated and in need of some inward direction. Continue to maintain your balance and share with others. If you have adapted skills that have allowed you to create peace and harmony in your life and career, I would like to salute you by doing a double-twist, backhanded somersault and letting out a loud, mezzo-soprano "whoo hoo!" I would like to encourage you to share your secrets with us. There can never be enough information out there to encourage and inspire us to awaken to who we truly are and to practice self-care. Thank you for being here with me, and remember that we should all stand in support of one another. If you need support in tapping that hidden potential you have to be a complete human being while nurturing yourself and others, you are in the right place to learn and grow.

Introduction

"Self-love, my liege, is not so vile a sin, as self-neglecting."
—WHKK H@ S@ DROD@D

I was watching a movie called "A Bug's Life" with my children one evening. In one of the funniest scenes, a bug-zapper light is attracting all sorts of flying critters. Mosquito #1 yells out to his friend, "Don't look at the light!" Mosquito #2 yells back in despair, "I can't help it!" Mosquito #2 had become so entranced by the light that he was rendered powerless and unable to exert any self-control. He was drawn right into the light, got zapped, and plummeted to the ground. Although Mosquito #1 was unsuccessful in preventing his friend's dreadful demise, he did what he could. It makes you wonder what power or strength he found within himself that prevented him from being destroyed by the bug-zapper as well. I asked my kids what they thought about it and they replied, "Mom, it's a cartoon. Don't be so serious!" Okay, I admit it. I can find profundity in the strangest places, but everything in life is fair game for learning.

As I see it, the nursing profession faces many challenges right now. Staff shortages, burnout, lack of resources, and many other things are impacting our profession. The quality of our patient care, the quality of our professional experiences, and the quantity/quality of life outside of work are also heavily impacted. People have different ways of dealing with hard times, and nurses are no exception. There are Mosquito #1's who know enough to stay out of the light, but not enough to convince others to do the same. There are Mosquito #2's who are in the dark, so to speak, and are so consumed by the darkness of transition that they seem to be headed for a downfall without even being cognizant of it. By grace, I am speaking from the position of Mosquito #1, yelling out to you, "Don't look at the light!" I hope my warning will be more effective and prevent you from going that way—I hope you will yell back, "Okay, I'm flying in another direction!"

WHAT THIS BOOK IS ABOUT

Nursing from the Inside-Out is not a book about patient care. There are thousands of books dedicated to the art of patient care. This book is not about sprinkling pixie dust on your problems and making them all better (but I could use some pixie dust if you have some to share!). This book is about caring for oneself, wholly and completely. Self-care ranges from honoring the choices you make that impact yourself personally, to the food you eat and the thoughts you think. The topic of self-care may be unfamiliar to some of you, especially if you are not involved in any type of holistic or complementary therapy practice, such as massage, Reiki, or acupuncture. In these modalities or healing practices, caring for the self is highly encouraged. This book is about transforming yourself and impacting your nursing practice through the art of self-care. Self-care is the conscious act of replenishing your body, mind, and spirit through various activities and rituals. This book is a summary of various self-care practices and tools derived from different holistic modalities and ancient healing practices. These tools can help you go from an angry mood to one of calmness by knowing which essential oil to use or which pressure point to touch to make the anger shift, or even by performing a simple breathing exercise that helps release the tension and makes way for compassion to flow. This book is about creating better ways to cope with the stressors and changes that occur daily in our lives. Many of the self-care practices and tools discussed in this book are actually more than meets the eye. Although many of these holistic practices may seem physical in nature, the final result is directed inward, within yourself. These practices have a history of being utilized for thousands of years and have very deep roots in health, well-being, and spirituality. The ultimate goal is to shift your outward focus on your patients, family, and other responsibilities to an inward focus on yourself.

Shifting to consider yourself as a priority may be a challenge initially, but I have faith in you. You will figure things out as your awareness allows you to, and in your own time. You are the queen or king of this book, and I am giving you permission to become the queen or king of your life. Each and every experience you have during our time together is for your personal/soul growth, well-being, and enlightenment. Because this book shares various modalities and provides you with exercises to practice, you can essentially design your own self-care routine and learn to manage your life from a point of clarity. The true essence of self-care is love. You will never be motivated to care for yourself completely unless you open your heart to you. One of my favorite slogans comes from those old L'Oréal commercials (I am dating myself here): "Because I'm worth it!" Self-care is never an issue when you know your true value. I am still exploring and adding to my self-worth daily (from the inside out). In *The Hidden Power of the Heart*, Sara Paddison said, "As you sincerely go for deeper levels of love, the results you'll have in well-being and increased quality of life will motivate you, leading you to a wider dimensional awareness. The results are so rewarding you can easily develop a passion for self-management." Basically, the road you take to self-care creates an endless journey to learning and self-awareness. Self-awareness is like a pair of glasses that allows us to see ourselves and the world differently. This is what allows us to live and nurse from the highest point of our consciousness. Ultimately, this is where the transformation takes place.

WHY I WROTE THIS BOOK

So why did I write this book? I wrote this book as a guideline to help others to better care for themselves and to learn about holistic modalities that can improve health and well-being. However, it also serves as a constant reminder to myself to maintain and model self-care on all levels of my being (body, mind, and spirit), and to inspire others to do the same. I wish I could show you a before-and-after picture of me (before and after I started practicing self-care), because you would be utterly amazed. Some of you who were familiar with the self-care-deprived version of "me" may read the rest of this book with your mouths open. Trust me, that is totally okay. My mouth was open part of the time when I was writing! The memory flashbacks to the person I used to be have left me thanking God for his grace and for giving me the ability to change from the inside out.

I can't show you a before-and-after picture, but I can give you an excerpt from "A Day in the Life of Rachel Before She Learned Self-Care, Self-Love, Self-Awareness, and So On." Don't be alarmed or embarrassed if you see some resemblance to yourself or a friend, because self-care deprivation can happen to anyone. In my not-so-distant past, I had many full, hectic days of caring for four darling, energetic children (all under the age of 10). Not only was I busy, I was tired and busy! If you look in the dictionary under the word "tired," you just might find a picture of me sleeping next to the definition! With four independent and curious children, I had to be organized and always prepared for the unknown. The way I attempted to survive during this period in my life was to get as much done for the next day as I possibly could, the night before. My schedule was so rigid, I could have bounced a quarter off of it. Between 5 and 6 p.m., I would leave work and pick my kiddies up from their daycare or after-school programs. We would discuss our victories and mishaps of the day, often enduring interruptions from restlessness and violations of each other's personal space. I could never understand how it is possible for four children in a minivan, with plenty of space, to always end up touching each other. Between 6 and 7 p.m., the children would gather around the table to finish their homework. This was my time to prepare dinner and debate the fact that Rice Crispy treats are neither a protein nor a vegetable. Those children who did not have homework were required to stay in the vicinity so that I could hear, smell, or see them. Sound strange? Let me explain. I can tell you, from past experience, that any time I have been unable to see my children in plain view, they have managed to physically alter themselves in some way. No major harm has come to them yet, but it would usually take more than 15 minutes to undo the mess they created. Celeste was the barber, who would cut patches out of her brothers' hair (when you least suspected she would). Cedric was the Sharpie-marker tattoo artist, who loved to leave permanent marks on visible places (like his face)! Chandler was usually the guinea pig for Celeste and

Cedric's innovative "fashion" concepts. I have taken pictures of him dressed up in a minimum of three Halloween costumes all at one time! Cheraé is another story. Being the eldest child, she has had the most amount of idle time alone. You know what they say: "An idle mind is the devil's playground." In this case, an idle mind was Cheraé's playground! I remember one day I was in the kitchen baking a pound cake, and she disappeared for about 15 minutes. My motherly senses kicked in and impressed a notion upon me to search for her. After quickly scanning our tiny apartment, I found her in the bathroom. Cheraé was standing stark naked and slicked down with Vaseline from head to toe. I screamed when I saw her and she screamed right back at me. When she let out her loud cry, the Vaseline that was thickly caked on her lips slowly slid into her mouth. She sounded like a muffled seal having an extremely bad day. Once I mentally established she was safe, I couldn't help but laugh at the mess she had gotten herself into. She has the biggest beautiful brown eyes I have ever seen, but you never would have known it with that thick film of Vaseline covering each of them, bilaterally! (The image always takes me back to the day she was born, when the nurse put erythromycin in her eyes.) I can't begin to tell you how many baths it took to get her degreased, or how many times she kept sliding from my hands. In the meantime, the fire alarm in the apartment began to go off and I realized that a potentially lovely pound cake had been seriously neglected and severely burnt when all was said and done. So you can clearly see how these sporadic "unforeseen" events made it necessary for me to keep tight reigns on my children's safety and my sanity.

Getting back to my story, one evening during supper I noticed that Celeste wasn't finishing her food. She was just sitting there. I didn't understand what her deal was, so I began my line of questioning. I learned that my daughter had decided to save her food that day because she didn't think there was enough for me to eat. I asked her why she thought that. She replied, "You never eat with us, Mommy." That moment was piercing. She wasn't eating because she was saving her food for me. When my kids were small, I never ate with them. I always watched them eat. I was usually too tired, wound up from the day, and had no appetite to eat at all once I finished cooking. I would stand watch at the kitchen table during meal times so I could refill milk glasses promptly, dish out second helpings, wipe mouths, and be on spill patrol when the need arose. I begin to reflect on the quality of the time I was able to spend with my children, in the midst of the hustle and bustle to get things completed. It wasn't very good. Our busy lives were nothing short of an assembly line in a factory (morning and night). I was a parent. I was just a worker doing my job to "get 'em up, fed, and out of the house. . . get 'em home, fed, and straight to bed!" Just as my daughter had her own perceptions, I had perceptions of life as I knew it to be. I know now that my perceptions weren't accurate, at that time, but they were very real for me then. My perception was that there wasn't enough time for me, because my children's primary needs came first, at all costs. But I wasn't meeting their primary needs like I thought I was. There was little quality in the quantity, because I was just trying to survive.

I am reminded of a story my psychology teacher shared once. Every Thanksgiving, a large family (at least three generations) would gather together, as many families do. In this family, it was customary to always have a big ham with the end cut off. One Thanksgiving, a little girl was watching her mother put a big ham in the baking pan, but first the mother cut off the end of the ham and put it to the side. The little girl innocently asked her mother why she did that. The mother didn't have a specific answer other than this was the way her mother always prepared the ham. That answer didn't satisfy the little girl, so she went to her grandmother. The grandmother's answer was pretty much along the same lines as her daughter's. The little girl wasn't satisfied with that answer either. Her final stop was her great-grandmother. The great-grandmother explained that she always served a big ham for the holiday, but her pan was too small for the ham. That was the only reason why she cut the end of the ham off. Cutting off the end imparted no magical flavors imparted to the ham whatsoever. The little girl observed how people will do things a certain way, without question, just because that's how it's always been done. We carry out the traditions we have learned in our personal lives and in nursing, oftentimes without question, because this is the way that things have always been done. If our traditions don't serve us and add to our lives and our growth, they are maladaptive. How will we ever know, unless we begin to listen to that little voice that asks, "Why?"

My daughter was that little voice of reason for me. She helped me to see the lingering of a tradition that was no longer needed. I don't remember my mother eating with us, but she was always there. She stood by the table waiting on us hand and foot until we were done. My grandmother did the same thing for her children, except that there were 10 of them. I was subconsciously acting out the same life I had lived as a child, the same life my mother lived as a child, and so on. I was impacted by my hectic schedule at work. I was serving my children. I was tired, needing to eat, and inevitably heading for some sick time.

Back to my story: Between 7 and 9 p.m., I would lay out clothes, pack lunches, line up book bags at the door, finish giving baths, make sure everyone said their prayers, and finally get the children tucked in. When 10 p.m. rolled around, I would be asleep before my head hit the pillow. My thoughts before falling to sleep were always related to the dread of having to get up and do it all again the next day. My worst fear was that one day I would wake up and not have the will or energy to get up and even make it through my workday.

What was my workday like? In case you were wondering, the time spent at work was no different from that at home. The perception I had of not having enough time to get everything done was exactly the same. I was trapped in a crazy cycle. Empty and tired, I was certain I had gotten into the wrong profession. I found myself feeling cynical, negative, and resentful inside because everyone was demanding so much of me all the time. I couldn't enjoy my children, because caring for them seemed to be a struggle. I couldn't enjoy my patients, because caring for them seemed to be a struggle too. I was caught in a vicious cycle of nurse/mother on the brink of a mega meltdown. I worked through lunches all the time and barely went to the restroom. I accepted every patient to my caseload who requested me, regardless of whether my schedule was full or not. Who was I to disappoint them? I did not want to disappoint my supervisors either. I had a severe case of guilt when I needed to say no. It was easier for me to just accept more responsibility, even though the little voice in the pit of my stomach was yelling at me to "step away from the patient, don't take that extra shift, check your calendar before you commit!" You can see how easy it is to head toward the light, entranced, when you live that type of existence.

HOW TO READ THIS BOOK

There is no incorrect way to read this book. You can read it alone or with a group. Reading alone is great because you can process and self-reflect in solitude. If you choose to read this book as part of a group, you and the other members can support one another in your efforts to overcome the daily challenges and stressors of nursing and of life. There may be many concepts that are new to you, but you are not required to understand everything immediately. Some things just unfold in their own time. Be open to not having all the answers, because I definitely don't. I just know what works for me, and you have to learn what works for you. The only thing you need to understand is that you deserve to care for yourself. You may have to read this book several times to incorporate various modalities into your life. You may be led to read other books that help you tie things together. You may learn a great deal, see progress in your outer world, and feel the changes in your inner self. By all means, celebrate your victories. Each day is a new experience and challenges come as opportunities to teach us lessons. You will get those lessons! If you find yourself reverting back to old ways of thinking, despite what you know is best for you, I implore you to be gentle and loving to yourself always.

WHO SHOULD READ THIS BOOK?

Any physician or healthcare professional is welcome to (and should) read this book and learn the art of self-care. The concepts apply to anyone who cares for others in any capacity. This book comes from my nursing experiences, so I see things from a nursing perspective. Nevertheless, if you aren't a nurse, you are still among friends. We can still support one another because we are in this together.

Every nurse should read this book because no one is exempt from experiencing burnout, compassion fatigue, hopelessness, powerlessness, illness, and spiritual distress from the stressors that exist in everyday life (home and work). It doesn't matter whether you already practice some form of self-care; if you think there's nothing more you can learn about it, you could be in for the surprise of your life.

More importantly, nursing students should read this book. Nursing programs can be stressful for anyone, but they can be especially difficult for the student who is trying to raise a family, work, and juggle school at the same time, as many are. Once that student walks across the graduation stage, his or her coping mechanisms may be nearly exhausted. But the stress doesn't stop, because there is the board exam. The stress doesn't stop after the board exam, because there is orientation. Any coping behaviors that were learned or practiced in a person's life are carried on to nursing school. These behaviors will surely carry over into the workforce, whether they are healthy or maladaptive. If students can begin to use self-care tools while they are in nursing school, they can lay the groundwork to be healthy and balanced as they embark upon a new and rewarding career.

Before we embark upon our journey, let me leave you with this thought: Wouldn't it be awesome if we could have a day set aside, nationally, that would allow nurses to celebrate self-care and self-nurturing freely? When I say "freely," I mean recognized by every employer and not considered optional. Every single nurse would take this day seriously and honor herself or himself by carrying out special self-care activities unique to his or her personal needs. As we see this vision growing, not only will nurses have this day off, they won't have to worry about covering their shifts. It would all be taken care of because the doctors would volunteer to pitch in and cover for them (they may need an orientation beforehand, but I have faith they can pull it off!). Wouldn't it be even greater if this National Self-Care Day extended to our homes and was honored by our family and friends? The icing on the cake would be to know that every single nurse in the world had his or her own daily self-care routine (outside of a national day) that he or she practices, consistently, to maintain balance and inner peace. I know all of this may seem farfetched (especially the part about doctors volunteering to take our shifts), but anything is possible. I can say "anything is possible" because I personally know many nurses who make self-care a part of their daily lives. I hear this can be very contagious. So let's get to spreading this behavior all over the place and create that world we have only dreamed about!

CHAPTER 1

The Importance of Self-Care for Nurses

RACHEL Y. HILL

*"The name of the game is taking care of yourself,
because you're going to live long enough to wish you had."*
—GRACE MIRABELLA

THE IMPORTANCE OF SELF-CARE FOR NURSES

Like a character in a romance novel, every nurse has a personal story explaining his or her passion for entering the nursing profession. Nursing school reflects a blissful courtship that allows the two (the student and the profession) to get acquainted with one another. The courtship is not without its stress, but the relationship advances. The engagement advances through the various years of study, and the pinning ceremony represents the commitment between the individual and the nursing profession. The job is the marriage that actually binds the two as one. Of course, there is a honeymoon period during which things seem to be perfect and the match made in heaven keeps one in a state of bliss. The things we do not particularly like in the other are tolerated because we have invested too much in the relationship to not be happy. In fact, we may have invested so much in the relationship that we no longer resemble who we used to be. There is not enough time. Taking care of the needs of nursing and the patients prevents us from having time for ourselves. The resentment increases because there is a feeling of entrapment. As sometimes happens in a marriage, the good times fluctuate and the bad times come more frequently. As time brings about changes, we begin to wonder, where did the love go? The individual has changed and the nursing profession has changed. No one seems to understand what happened. They seem to have outgrown each other, with nothing left in common but a picture of a ceremony uniting the two as one. A once beautiful romance story has dwindled away before our own eyes.

HISTORY OF SELF-CARE

Self-care is a concept that has been around for thousands of years, but has probably been referred to as something as simple as "rest." The day of God's rest

1

has long since evolved into a day of rest and worship called the Sabbath. Many religions observe the Sabbath. The term "observance" usually means to totally refrain from daily activities and work. Genesis 2:2 in the Bible states that after the completion of 7 days of work, God saw fit to take a rest. "By the seventh day God completed His work which He had done, and He rested on the seventh day from all His work which He had done."

Outside of religious observances, Friday through Saturday can be a time in which people become anxious and geared up. Parties, camping trips, and weekend getaways are some of the things that are reserved for the "weekend" or days of rest. It is not by coincidence that the excitement of the weekend has led to acronyms like TGIF, because at the end of each week people anticipate the rest and relaxation they will enjoy after all their hard work. As you can see, historically, self-care has been incorporated into our life through religious and cultural means. I remember not too long ago, when I was a little girl, the city stores would shut down early on Saturday and be closed on Sunday. It's amazing how times have changed. The weekend resembles a regular day of the week because people don't rest on the weekends and businesses stay open to make money.

Some of the greatest minds in history have left behind their wisdom in literature, encouraging others to take the time to love, care, and think of themselves with the highest regard. We can clearly see how self-care was just as important hundreds of years ago as it is to us today. François de la Rochefoucauld (1613–1680), a French Classical author, once said, "Self-love is the greatest of all flatterers." Benjamin Franklin (1706–1790) once said, "He that falls in love with himself, has no rivals." William Henry Davies (1871–1940) wrote a poem entitled "Leisure":

Leisure

What is this life if, full of care,
We have no time to stand and stare.
No time to stand beneath the boughs
And stare as long as sheep or cows.
No time to see, when woods we pass,
Where squirrels hide their nuts in grass.
No time to see, in broad daylight,
Streams full of stars, like skies at night.
No time to turn at Beauty's glance,
And watch her feet, how they can dance.
No time to wait till her mouth can
Enrich that smile her eyes began.
A poor life this is if, full of care,
We have no time to stand and stare.

The history of self-care can also be found in various healing practices that have been around for centuries. Jin Shin Jyutsu, or Japanese acupressure, means the art of knowing oneself. A strong emphasis is placed on the individual who is receiving Jin Shin Jyutsu to become proficient in his or her own self-care through learned practices. In the first level of Reiki, a Japanese form of energy medicine, the students learn to care for themselves before setting out to help others. In the 1970s, the Therapeutic Touch program was begun by Doris Kunz and Delores Krieger. This nurse-based modality encouraged nurses to not only share energy work with patients, but to work on the self as well. In the mid-1970s, Jean Watson (a nursing theorist) created a significant theory that considered the self-care needs of the caregiver/nurse along with the needs of the patient. This relationship had not been explored in a theory before that time.

In the early 1980s, the American Holistic Nurses Association (AHNA) was founded by Charlotte McGuire, with five core values of holistic nursing. One of the five core values is self-care for the holistic nurse. This organization has been the springboard for the endorsement of many programs, literature, and research relating to holistic practices for patient care, nurturing of nurses, and creating a holistic consciousness among nurses worldwide. Not only do nurses begin to understand how to care for patients holistically, they also begin to recognize the value of understanding their strengths and weaknesses, personally and professionally. The ability to reflect on independent beliefs, thoughts, actions, and interactions with others can help lead to a great self-awareness.

In the 1990s, the Healing Touch program was started by Janet Mentgen with the help of other nurses and the AHNA, with the heart of the practice being self-care for the nurse/healer. The nurse as a healer is supported and encouraged to practice self-care in all aspects of his or her life, to maintain vitality and the ability to reach out to others. The Healing Touch program and Healing Touch International are extensions of Janet Mentgen's vision, and its members continue to educate new Healing Touch students, nurses who practice the healing touch modality, and lay people in healing-based modalities both locally and internationally.

Currently the AHNA, Healing Touch International, Healing Touch Program, American Nurses Association (ANA), and many state boards and organizations are at the forefront in supporting nursing programs that promote the concept of self-care for achieving balance in all aspects of life.

EVOLUTION OF HEALTH CARE

Today we call allopathic medicine "traditional medicine," although it was not the first traditional form of health care available to us. All other forms of medicine are in the category of "alternative" or "complementary." However, the roots of allopathic medicine can be traced back to nature (the first traditional medicine) and its interactions with the body, mind, and spirit as a whole. As science began to prevail in the early 20th century, René Descartes perceived the need to protect the conscious mind from the corruption of the growing force of science. The body could be left to the exploration of science. It would be the responsibility of the church to tend to the mind and spirit of man. Although his intentions were noble, it led to a separation between treatment of the body and the whole person (Koopsen & Young, 2009). During this time, the belief evolved that the mind has no major correlation with disease. The second era of medicine occurred in the 1950s, when the mind was still considered separate from the body but became of more interest in relation to a person's consciousness. People began to discover that the mind does indeed have a connection with the body. In the third era of medicine, we have learned to believe in the connection between consciousness and the body (and beyond), and experience our connection with our inner selves and with others. Numerous modalities, such as prayer, healing touch, reiki, and shamanism (Dossey & Keegan, 2009), are used. These practices often complement allopathic medicine and may not be customary in religious practices; however, they are at the forefront in bringing us to a new level of healing for ourselves (body, mind, and spirit). As we discuss self-care, we will look at ways that allow us to integrate all aspects of caring and healing into our being.

Impact of Healthcare Changes for Nurses

Table 1-1   Twenty-five Reasons for Practicing Self-Care

1. You fall asleep in your scrubs.
2. You fall asleep in your garage, because you never make it from your car into your house.
3. You can't remember driving home.
4. Your wardrobe consists of scrubs only and you wear them to weddings, graduations, baptisms, church services, barmistvas, etc.)
5. You answer your home phone and unit/office phone the same way.
6. Your lunch consists of graham crackers, juice, and cheese from the diabetic's snack stash.
7. You work a 12 hour shift without ever needing to take a restroom break.
8. You feel betrayed when your coworker is leaving you to take a family vacation.
9. Every lunch is always a working lunch.
10. People on the day shift think you work nights.
11. People on the night shift think you work days.
12. You sleep with your pager and/or cellphone under your pillow.
13. You are so tired that you put your laptop in the refrigerator by accident.
14. Your patients refer you to their psychologists for antidepressants.
15. You use your nursing diploma as a dart board for recreation.
16. Your lap has formed indentions from the laptop always resting there.

17. You consider your daily 8 ozs. of fluid to be cups of coffee or coke.
18. You are styling your hair and use spray starch instead of the hairspray.
19. You take a sick day rather than work a shift with a certain coworker.
20. People scatter when you approach their area.
21. Your thoughts about your patients or coworkers cannot be repeated out loud (without disciplinary action).
22. All your hobbies and pastimes are nursing related.
23. You take home the "most overtime" award every single year.
24. Your idea of a massage is the smooth side of the plastic back scratcher or urinal.
25. You send sympathy cards to graduates from the nursing program you have precepted.

What Is Self-Care?

Before we can establish the importance of self-care for nurses, we must first determine what self-care is. Self-care is the means by which individuals replenish their mental, physical, and spiritual beings through conscious action. This means of action is often holistic in nature and often comes from complementary and alternative therapies. According to the AHNA, there are three categories of self care practices: a *physical* category, an *emotional/spiritual* category, and an *intellectual* category. The physical category of self-care relates to any physical activity that one might undertake to promote a healthy lifestyle. Exercising to stay fit, practicing good nutrition to maintain health, hugging trees, planting a garden, salsa dancing, and getting a massage to minimize stress are all physical means that contribute to maintaining balance. The second category of self-care, the emotional/spiritual category, relates to practices that connect you with yourself and with others, and help you tap into something greater than what you can physically experience. Daily prayer and devotions, a meditative practice, Qi Gong, Tai Chi, various forms of yoga, keeping a journal, nature walks, and music therapy are all practices that can shift your emotional and spiritual consciousness for the better. The third category of self-care practice is the intellectual category. You are actually engaged in that category now, because you are reading this book! Reading books, taking classes for fun or for continuing education, and listening to compact discs or tapes are ways in which you can engage your intellect and expand your self-awareness.

Terminology Relating to Self-Care

Burnout – A syndrome prone to caregivers that is caused by mental, emotional, and physical stressors that create conditions of tension and detachment within the caregiver in the everyday dealings with the clients that he or she works with.

Compassion fatigue – The depletion in the reserves of compassion that a caregiver is able to exhibit for the clients cared for on a day-to-day basis, due to stressors that impact the caregiver.

Self-care deprivation – Self-care deprivation is the failure to meet one's self-care needs because of a lack of education or physical/mental/emotional/spiritual constraints.

Stress – The term "stress" refers to mental, emotional, and physical stimuli that pose a threat to an individual's well-being.

Why Self-Care Is Important to Nurses

Self-care helps us restore balance and neutralize the challenges or stressors we face in life, and maintain our balance within. When we think of the importance of self-care in nursing, we can easily compare it with our regularly scheduled car maintenance, annual physicals, and tasks such as mowing the lawn and cleaning the gutters. These activities are routine and fairly simple. Difficulties can result when we don't keep up with our scheduled routines. Don't service your car and you may eventually have problems with a number of things—your tires, engine, alternator, and battery are just a few things that can suffer from neglect and cost many dollars down the road. Don't have an annual physical and one or more of your systems (endocrine, nervous, digestive system, etc.) may eventually require a special procedure, medication, or test because of your negligence. Don't mow your lawn and you will end up with a jungle that attracts an entire animal kingdom to live there (and only animal control can help you get rid of it!). House maintenance can be another nightmare, should you fail to do your part as a homeowner. Being diligent in maintenance means being responsible and paying attention to the things in our lives that have the potential to break down or deteriorate over time. Self-care maintenance is no different; it requires us to be responsible by paying attention to our body, mind, spirit, home, career, and relationships with ourselves and others. The things that often get in the way of what is most important to us are stress and time. A wise person once said an ounce of prevention is worth a pound of cure. Self-care is definitely a pound of cure.

There is much publicity about what is wrong with the nursing profession these days. However, the risks nurses face and the challenges they endure are worth mentioning. Facing the challenges openly will help us to move forward and address those challenges consciously. With all the transitions the healthcare profession faces, it would be very easy to take the low road and focus on what we lack instead of on what we truly have as a profession. Let's look at what we have as a profession first, before we look at what we don't have. What do we have as a profession? I recently attended a brunch and listened to Wendy Wright, a nurse practitioner, discuss pediatric skin diseases. In her introduction, she noted that she had her own practice with nurse practitioners, with 38 on staff and almost 1200 patients. She and a colleague had created a company that provides education for nurse practitioners free of charge, through grants. I was in awe! This is what is good about nursing. I know there are more dynamic people just like her. Once she began to talk about skin diseases, however, I thought I might have a hard time being entertained. I had no idea that anyone could keep me on the edge of my seat by simply talking about skin diseases. But while she was talking to the group about scabies, I was hanging on to every word. She made it just that exciting to me! Her knowledge on the topic was incredible, her delivery style was humorous and energetic, and the contributions she had made to nursing were absolutely remarkable. I had a strong sense that nursing was truly her calling and passion, because from the events she described that were going on in her life, things just seemed to be falling in place for her. I just had a hunch she was definitely meant to be a nurse practitioner. What I often see in our profession is a natural ability to facilitate healing in others, by so many means. Our ability to educate creates the opportunity to change the lives of patients and colleagues every day. The ability nurses have to be at the forefront of patient care gives us the opportunity to save lives over and over again.

What do we lack in our profession? From a statistical standpoint, plain and simple, we are lacking nurses. The Nursing Shortage Fact Sheet, produced by the American Association of Colleges of Nursing states that "the shortage of registered nurses in the U.S. could reach as high as 500,000 by 2025 according to a report released by Dr. Peter Buerhaus and colleagues in March 2008." The report, entitled "The Future of the Nursing Workforce in the United States: Data, Trends, and Implications," found that the demand for RNs is expected to grow by 2% to 3% each year" (www.jbpub.com/catalog/9780763756840). According to Donley (2005), we have 80% of 2.8 million nurses practicing in the United States. Many of the nurses who are currently working are not what I would call "full-strength" nurses. These nurses are diluted by the transitions of health care, the economy, and the residual effects of the nursing shortage. I haven't even begun to throw in the personal challenges of family, finances, health, or other obstacles outside the work setting. These nurses are not currently experiencing their maximum potential as human beings, let alone as nurses. There is a law called the Universal Law of Attraction. The basis of this law is that what we give our attention to on a daily basis mentally, emotionally, and physically, we will attract into our lives. It doesn't surprise me that we are unable to attract more nurses to the workforce, to retain nurses in the workforce, or to maintain our satisfaction in the workforce. We have nurses in the workforce who are not satisfied with their careers. "The challenging composition of the nursing workforce and the dissatisfaction of practicing nurses contribute to the complexity of the nursing shortage" (Donley, 2005).

Nurses are valuable assets in all healthcare settings and in the community. The theme I keep uncovering is that this is not so much unrealized by the employer and patients as it is unrealized by the nurses themselves. How can you be appreciated or expect to be appreciated by your employers when you don't realize that you are something special? I have to admit that there are some environments in which you will never get feedback and may have to ask the question, Do I make a difference here? If you cannot see your worth, and your self-esteem is being pulverized, I would say it is time to move to a healthier environment and work on mending your wings. The nurse has to be strong and have a sense of their own value to even begin honoring himself or herself in ways that he or she deserves. That strong sense of self doesn't come overnight. If you don't learn to establish a strong sense of self, you will begin to look for external satisfaction through compliments, praise, rewards, and public displays of gratitude for services rendered. If you don't receive these outer strokes for the ego, you will begin to feel dissed! When you feel dissed, you will feel dismayed, disappointed, disgruntled, diseased, and dissatisfied as a result of your lack of self-esteem. My grandfather used to say, "You have to know that you know that you know. . . ." You have to know that you know that you are a good nurse; otherwise, your service to others will be superficial and you will need external means to motivate you to help others. Nursing should come from a much deeper place; otherwise, all your efforts will be futile.

I know a nurse who is the best home-health nurse I have ever met. She is creative and gifted, and inspires her patients to do some pretty remarkable things. She once had a patient who was at risk for losing his legs because of horrible skin ulcers. This nurse educated the family, motivated them and the patient, and was able to help save the patient's legs. I was talking to her and sharing my observations with her about her sensitivity to her patients. I was her manager and wanted to express to her that her presence and abilities were priceless. It wasn't until later, when she and I talked, that she told me she thought I was patronizing her. And yet I was so sincere, and held such a high regard for her as a nurse. I don't think she had really stopped to think how awesome she was! It was only later that I learned about many challenging experiences she had with other managers, and so many moments in which she had felt unappreciated. I understood why my encouragement felt like something else to her.

Self-care is important to nursing because the preservation of the nursing profession is dependent on it. The nurse's self-awareness will be the very state that allows him or her to take responsibility for conditions in the workplace and in the home environment. The well-being of each individual nurse will determine the state of the nursing profession because it is the nurse's ability to nurture himself or herself that allows them to care for patients effectively and with compassion. Although it has been stated that nurses who work in hospital settings are more challenged and stressed than nurses who work in other settings, it must be realized that all nurses are exposed to tremendous amounts of stress in the workforce.

Let's quickly review stress and its impact on the body. There are many definitions of stress. Stress is the felt experience of overactivity of the sympathetic nervous system (Dossey & Keegan, 2009). According to Koopsen and Young (2009), stress is the reaction to any stimulus or challenge that upsets our normal function and disturbs our mental or physical health.

My Personal Story

My first informal introduction to self-care was observing our Sabbath as a day of rest and watching my father. We did absolutely nothing on Sunday, because my mother worked diligently to cram everything in on the night before. She cooked, cleaned, ironed, and did everything to keep from lifting a finger on Sunday. The Sabbath was also a day of worship for us. My grandfather was the pastor for a rapidly growing church, so my family was very active in serving others all the time. Our Sabbath wasn't just on Sunday. It seemed as if it fell on every day of the week. I served in many capacities—I was an usher, I sang in the choir, I served on the hospitality committee, I was a Sunday-school president, and I worked on the nursing board. There were always people to visit in their home or nursing home, or in the hospital. There was always a family to comfort and a funeral to attend. My grandfather was always on the go and was on call 24/7. My grandparents, uncles, aunts, and parents sacrificed a great deal of their time and many opportunities to do other things, because the ministry and service to God were the most important things to them at that time. Working in the church is definitely a labor of love and calls for much sacrifice. Serving others was what I knew. The idea of self-care would have made me very uncomfortable, and would have seemed selfish. I was so used to serving others in any capacity I could, it was difficult to have down time when I wasn't serving others. If I wasn't serving others, I would find someone who needed me somewhere, because self-care wasn't in my frame of reference at that time.

I learned about self-care from watching my father every evening after work. I thought it was a "man thing." Applying what I now know about self-nurturing to my image of his actions then, I realize that he practiced his self-care perfectly. When he came home from work every day, he went straight to his velvety green recliner. He would put up his feet, and one of my brother or sisters would help take off his shoes. He would read his newspaper, watch the news, have a cold glass of Pepsi, and wait for dinner. We would take his dinner to him on a tray. We would take his tray when he was done. Sometimes I would catch him dosing, but I knew not to disturb him. You might think it would be hard to keep five children quiet, but it wasn't. We knew better than to make a peep when dad first got home. He needed time to unwind because he worked so hard to provide for us. My mother made sure that we had a clear understanding of this. Of course, my dad didn't argue one bit. He expected nothing less from us, because he valued himself and took pride in being the sole provider for his family. He would play basketball, work out at the YMCA, go fishing, play the guitar, and listen to his George Benson albums. My father may have taken the concept of self-care a little to the extreme, but I can assure you that we weren't his indentured servants. I never saw my mother take a vacation, have a girls' night out, or anything like that. Her life revolved around her family. Dad was the king of his castle and my mother was the perfect housewife, catering to her husband and raising her children. As a female, I would grow up to do the same.

My first formal introduction to the concept of self-care was in a Jin Shin Jyutsu class in 1998. I had graduated from nursing school in 1996, but I don't think self-care was discussed in enough detail for me to remember. I wish we had practiced self-care as much as we prepared for boards. I might have adjusted a little better to my surroundings. Perhaps I was taught about self-care, but the stress of being a new graduate was so intense, I just forgot everything I was taught. I attended a religion-based nursing school and was fortunate to have a spiritual outlet during nursing school. Our class shared in devotions and prayer before each class and clinical rotation, and we were able to begin our day with a spiritual focus. As a graduate of a Nazarene college and the grandchild of a pastor, if I knew how to do anything at all, it was how to pray!

Once I graduated from nursing school, I was ready to serve others. I found myself blindsided by the many unforeseen challenges that my nursing program had not prepared me for. The biggest issues I faced in my first year of nursing were an unsupportive nursing environment ("eating the young"), mandatory overtime, and not being able to begin the actual orientation until 3 months after I began work. Whether I asked questions, didn't ask questions, or "knew too much," I always found myself in some sort of trouble. After surviving a shift, I felt like I had a gnawed limb hanging off my body. After less than 6 months of working as a nurse, my dreams of a glorious career started to fade. This was when feelings of insecurity and powerlessness, unhealthy internalizing, and a tiny seed of the idea that I should leave nursing began to grow. It's hard to keep those types of feelings from reaching home. I had my own visions of how I should be as a mother and as a wife. I knew I was smart, but as a new nurse, I felt like nothing was looking like it did in the textbooks. I didn't have the time to assimilate anything. My expectations of myself were high, but my performance wasn't matching what I hoped it would be. Poor coping skills, an exhausted mental capacity, and low morale left me unable to maintain a marriage with four children to raise. Prayer was the only self-care I had ever practiced. After enduring enough conflicts and receiving little support, though, I couldn't even form a prayer with my lips.

My self-care practices were highly influenced by the ways in which I was raised. My gender, religious beliefs, and cultural experiences played a very important part in how I was able to accept and practice self-care. With nursing being a service-oriented profession, it is so easy for me to regress to the totally natural feeling of complete service to others. My expectations to perform as my mother did were unrealistic. I was a full-time mother, wife, and employee, and had a little bit more on my plate than she had. I had so much guilt over the fact that I couldn't do it all, and I began to berate myself over and over. I didn't stop trying, though, and eventually learned to let go of the guilt, but these embedded habits are hard to break. If you let your guard down one bit, you begin to resemble that old person you thought had gone to rehab and recovered. This is when self-care for me becomes most important and I have to practice balance. I have an internal mechanism inside that goes off when I am out of balance. I begin to feel edgy and trapped, and the natural flow of things begins to become laborious and forced. This is when I step back, reevaluate, and practice self-care to reestablish my equilibrium.

Impact of Stress

There are two types of stressors: good and bad. Good stress, of course, is experienced when we win the lottery, get married, get promoted, win a carnival prize, or get surprised with flowers. Examples of bad stress include when we experience the death of a loved one, life's challenges, and extremely large bills. Whether the stressors are good or bad, though, over a prolonged period of time, the effects may cause changes in the body that can lead to illness. When one is faced with an impossible workload, staffing that is inadequate and unsafe, conflicting relationships with coworkers, insufficient time to complete work, micromanagers, powerlessness to achieve outcomes, lack of team work, lack of administrative support, inability to meet a patient's emotional needs, and ongoing issues involving trauma, death, and dying, one can easily see why self-care is so important to nursing. These types of stress, over a prolonged period of time, can have a significant impact on our mental and emotional states, eventually causing physical illness as well.

No challenge we face in life externally will ever be resolved solely by physical means. There will always be an internal drive, a moment of enlightenment, a bright idea, and a conviction that spills forth, is put into action, and is manifested in the world to create a resolution. Articles on the challenges of nursing, committees for retention of nurses, and surveys of opinions and attitudes provide us with a snapshot of the climate. Self-care gives us the ability to tune into ourselves and cause meaningful changes that can transform our climate. As we transform, our focus changes, allowing the law of attraction to help us create a new and exciting workforce. "Thought is cause!" If you don't like your job, don't try to recruit others. If all your conversations are about what is wrong with nursing, stop complaining about what is wrong—you have just reinforced that image even more. Sister Rosemary Donley (2005) calls this "negative nursing affectivity." We use the negatives of nursing to try to convince people of what we need, because things are so bad. A side effect of that is that we end up putting a poor image of nursing out into the world, resulting in the perception that we are victims or mentally deficient. We don't deny the challenges we face, but we can face those challenges responsibly by caring for ourselves appropriately. The same precision and perfection that we offer our patients should be the same care we offer to ourselves. Why? Because we deserve everything good life has to offer us. If things that seem bad come our way, we deserve to have resources to handle those things with grace and ease! In nurturing ourselves, we can create positive nursing affectivity. We can make conscious choices to take our experiences of work overload, lack of resources, and stress, and transform them into something more powerful than the issue itself. The only way to do this is by nurturing yourself, which changes your thoughts, which changes your reality, which allows you to respond differently to situations, which promotes growth.

ASSESSING YOUR NEED FOR SELF-CARE

Table 1-2 is a Self-Care Questionnaire that will help you to determine more in detail where you stand on the self-care spectrum. There are no ratings or scales. Simply read the questions, answer the questions, and then read the questions and answers back to yourself. Spend some time and sit with your answers. If it turns out that you are in need of lots of self-love, don't throw yourself into a pit of guilt. We will get you headed in the right direction.

Table 1-2   Self-Care Questionnaire

1. Does the thought of going to work the next day cause physical discomfort for you?
2. Do you feel like everyone is against you? (staff, patients, family).
3. Do you have a balance between work and home life?
4. Do you provide care for others outside of the workplace?
5. Do you take care of yourself, before you take care of others?
6. Do feel like your work demands are intense, but don't stop when you get home?
7. Do you like the environment you work in?
8. Do you like the people you work with and feel appreciated by them?
9. Do you have a supportive family (parents, husband, children)?
10. Do you have supportive coworkers?
11. Do you have hobbies and things you do for fun when you are not working?
12. Do you suffer from depression?
13. Are you physically out of shape and/or physically ill.
14. Do you miss out on family functions and outings because you are always at work?
15. When was the last time you had a home-cooked meal.
16. Do you anger or cry easily?

Theories to Consider

Yin-Yang Theory

I hope time will, one day, allow me to study Chinese medicine in depth, because I have a great appreciation for the contributions that herbal medicine and theories regarding the elements and balance can make in one's life. I see the influence of Chinese medicine in many of the modalities I practice. I transpose those theories to my life experience so that I can understand them better and learn from them. The theory of Yin-Yang is one of those contributions I am constantly drawing from in my daily life. Traditional Chinese medicine utilizes the theory of Yin-Yang as a unique means of viewing and treating the physical body, and the roots of this theory are more than 2000 years old.

The basic premise behind the Yin-Yang theory is the unity of opposites. For people in ancient times, the words Yin and Yang were used primarily to indicate whether a place was facing the sun's light. Yang described the place that faced the sunlight or was filled with sun. Yin described the place that faced away from the sunlight. These places of light and darkness are opposites of each other and created the basis for yin and yang. Today, the theory of Yin-Yang evolved to mean much more than light and darkness. The main aspects of Yin and Yang are that they are opposites. Things in our natural world have two opposite aspects. We have hot and cold, fire and water, male and female, soft and hard, etc. The opposites are dependent on each other for existence. The relationship between these aspects promotes change and development in our world. Life exists because even while this opposition is occurring, balance is maintained at the same time. There is a mutual consumption of Yin-Yang. Each opposite has a certain degree of the other, which enables ongoing change. The seasons are a perfect example of the graceful change we see at any given time of the year. Once winter is over, spring comes, then summer comes, then fall comes, and the cycle continues. The seasons consume each other in a mutual and natural way. One season doesn't come fully until the other has totally ended; however, there is a transition that occurs. It is like a shift change. No nurse will leave her shift without giving her report to the nurse who will take her place. They are both there for a time, exchanging information and asking questions of each other. The nurse leaves her notes, medicine administration record (MAR), and any other information that may be pertinent to the patients' care, and is finally free to go (i.e., until her season arrives again).

There are situations in which imbalance can occur, even though balance is the natural tendency. Say, for instance, the nurse had an emergency and wasn't available to give her report. The nurse assuming the shift would have questions and would not be able to proceed with her shift (or season) naturally. Things might be rocky at first, but things might eventually level out and the season would return to normalcy. Perhaps the nurse would be able to come back and share the information he or she needed to after the emergency was over, or maybe a supervisor or someone else would have enough information to be helpful in the transition, so that the shift could go smoothly. With the threat of global warming, the seasons may come prematurely and cause issues for farmers and natural habitats. An imbalance can arise from too much or too little Yin or Yang. These opposite aspects must have a mutual relation and mutual opposition in order for them to exist.

For the purposes of self-care, we will picture Yin as our personal life and work as our Yang. The fulfillment of our existence here on Earth has everything to do with how these sides (opposites) function. When we go to work, we always have a little "home" in us, and when we go home, we always have enough "work" in us to keep an equilibrium established. A smooth cycle should flow. The season changes when we leave home and go to work, and then the season changes again when we return back home. When we experience changes at work, such as a new boss, more patients, or changes in hours, we are faced with the risk that our equilibrium will be thrown off. When we experience changes at home, such as a marriage, pregnancy, divorce, death, or relocation, we face the same risk. Our careers often come with the responsibility of having to carry a pager, a cell phone, or Blackberry, or having a computer that can access all of the office files at a moment's notice. There is little time to feel like you have ever really gotten away from work. The same is true when you have a sick child at home and no one to cover your shift. You probably spend so much time worrying about that sick child that your work suffers, from more of the Yin being in the Yang place. One of our opposing sides becomes more dominant, and imbalance occurs. This imbalance can lead to a breakdown in our environment and ourselves if we do not know how to restore balance.

Maslow's Hierarchy of Needs

Abraham Maslow gave us a "hierarchy of needs" that stems from his psychological theory of human motivation (Van Wagner). Figure 1-1 illustrates the pyramid that is usually depicted to describe Maslow's hierarchy of needs. There are five levels, with the base of pyramid being the fifth level of physiological needs. The physiological needs consist of eating, sleeping, activity, and interaction with others and the environment. The fourth level is safety needs or our need to feel safe and protected from hurt, harm, or danger. The third level is the need to feel love and a sense of belonging, which includes friendship, associations, and partnerships with others. The second level of needs includes the "esteem needs," which consist of self-worth, self-respect, and self-esteem, and the ability to be autonomous and independent in the world. The first level is the self-actualization of needs, which allows us to exist at our full potential as individuals.

Figure 1-1   Maslow's hierarchy of needs.

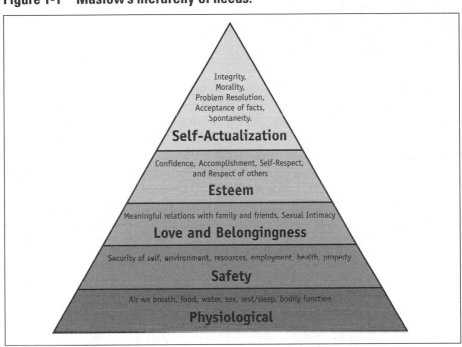

Integrity,
Morality,
Problem Resolution,
Acceptance of facts,
Spontaneity.

Self-Actualization

Confidence, Accomplishment, Self-Respect,
and Respect of others

Esteem

Meaningful relations with family and friends, Sexual Intimacy

Love and Belongingness

Security of self, environment, resources, employment, health, property

Safety

Air we breath, food, water, sex, rest/sleep, bodily function

Physiological

Source: © One02/ShutterStock, Inc.

According to Maslow, levels five to three consist of "deficit" needs (or D-needs), which result from deprivation. When you feel these needs are not being met, you attempt to fill them. There may be anxiety in your attempts to meet these needs. Each level builds on itself. If the first level is not met, you cannot experience the next level. The upper level needs are called growth or "being" needs (B-needs). These needs do not evolve from deprivation or a lack of something, but from the desire to reach one's highest potential as an individual. When we apply this hierarchy to nurses and the practice of nursing, we must remember that we are humans first before we are nurses. The needs we have as human beings for self-actualization can be transposed to our nursing careers because we want to reach self-actualization as nursing professionals just as we meet our physical needs for air, food, activity, etc. Our working environments must be comfortable, with proper heating and ventilation, for us to perform our jobs. Safety and protection needs must also be met. We must feel that we are safe when we're traveling to and from our patients' homes, when we're in our healthcare settings, and when we're working with patients and staff. The need for love and belongingness we have in the workplace is similar to the meaningful relationships we want to build at home with our families and our children. The teamwork approach, and knowing that another nurse "has your back" when you are in need, can make this level attainable. The need for esteem in the workplace is not just about feeling warm and fuzzy—it is about the worth that nurses feel regarding their jobs and themselves. Environments can be draining and seem not user-friendly. Administrators and managers can be good at informing nurses about what is wrong, and not so good at telling them what is right. This can make a nurse feel inadequate or unappreciated. Once the nurse has met the needs of this level and found ways to achieve self-certainty, he or she can move on to being the "super nurse." This is not to be confused with the nurse who tries to do it all. This is more like the nurse who has the capacity to do it all, because he or she is expansive but also knows the limits of healthy living and is able to balance life as a human being and as a nurse.

By applying the theory of Yin and Yang and the knowledge of Maslow's hierarchy, we can visualize the relationship between the worlds we must exist in every single day. We have lives outside of our work settings, and we have work outside our life settings. We must be able to balance both settings, and our needs must be met in both settings so that we can achieve inner peace and fulfill the individual potential that makes us the best we can be.

How Self-Care Impacts the Body

Let me try to describe the impact of self-care on the body to make it easier to understand from an energetic standpoint why self-care is needed. As humans, we are made up of three basic parts: body, mind, and spirit. We have emotions and thoughts generating internal stimuli that have the potential to cause stress. Our environment contains external stimuli that also have the potential to cause stress. Every human being has an "aura" or an energy field that surrounds his or her body. This field surrounds the body like an oval and contains a great deal of information that describes a person's physical, emotional, and spiritual states. The internal and external stimuli are in constant contact with our auric field, impacting it in random proportions. Internal stimuli that cause stress include our thoughts (which lead to emotions, which lead to reactions), illness, and pain. External stimuli that cause stress include problems, job challenges, deaths, and financial issues. If we are having a bad day, we are probably attracting more negative stimuli and creating more negative internal stimuli that weaken the aura further. On good days, we do just the opposite. Self-care consists of the acts that we do to support the body, mind, and spirit. There are different types of self-care that impact and nourish each category of our body. Self-care serves to buffer our bodies from the internal and external stimuli that can lead to stress. It serves to reinforce the auric field and rushes to the field to repair, neutralize, and reinforce any damage that internal and external stimuli stand to cause. Consider stress as a free radical that tears up the cellular membrane and causes damage. Consider self-care as an antioxidant that promotes healing and helps to buffer the effects that might cause something more detrimental farther down the line. Self-care does not prevent negative things from happening, but it can help one to adjust and neutralize more quickly.

Determining Your Order of Change

First-Order Change

I have shared with you reasons why self-care is important for your well-being. However, you might not consider them a sufficient motivation to change. I studied acupressure for 3 years, working diligently with others while practicing self-care once in a blue moon. One day, I read an article in *AHNA Beginnings* entitled *Caring for the Self: Becoming a Healing Presence* by Veda Andrus (2005), in which she discusses how nurses can create a healing presence for patients by practicing self-care in their own lives and explains orders of change. First-order changes are changes that we do because we read that we should or someone else tells us we should, or we might see someone else doing something interesting we want to try. These changes are short-term or superficial, and don't have long-lasting impacts on our lifestyle because our old coping mechanisms kick back in and prevent us from making a lasting change. Let's take my daily habit of flossing for example. I realized that I had been flossing with a first-order mentality. It was first order for me because it was something I had always been told to do. I had flossed whenever the mood hit me or I was annoyed by something obvious in between my teeth.

Second-Order Change

A shift in one's ability to be consistent is a second-order change. Second-order change is the change that carries more weight and has deeper connections with our intentions. We think less about why we should do things and begin to reframe or explore the values of the changes we are considering. When I had the threat of a cavity, I decided within myself that I wanted to keep my teeth for as long as I could. I decided that not flossing was irresponsible and not honoring myself. I have the power to maintain healthy teeth, and not doing so would be going against myself. This change was more experiential for me (Andrus, 2005). I have had cavities before, but this experience was different. This time I had the power to make a real change. All the things I have learned about self-care up to now caused the simple act of flossing to resonate differently with me because I was more aware of my needs and had a true desire to care for myself.

The ultimate goal is for nurses to implement self-care from a second-order change. What could make such an awesome change possible? You feel fine now because you are strong-willed and have a great amount of determination that keeps you going, or because you are from good genetic stock, and physical demands don't phase you because you're used to handling a great deal of pressure. Perhaps as a child you developed the ability to function under mental pressure; in fact, that may seem to be the only way you like to get things done. Whatever your scenario, coping strategy, or physical makeup, life has an amazing way of bringing about change within us and without us. The most important part is how we are able to respond to the changes that occur. If I could eat all the carbohydrates now that I ate as a kid, and not gain any weight, I would pitch a tent at my local Panera Bakery. No one is stopping me from eating bagels and pastries every day, but I have a deeper awareness of the changes my body has made over time. I choose to be conscious of them.

I find storms so amazing because of the impact they have on nature. When I see branches all over the ground after a storm, it doesn't faze me nearly as much as seeing a big oak tree ripped from the ground and lying in the middle of a yard. How could something so strong, with roots planted so deep, be plucked from the ground like a daisy? I am sure the tree was just as surprised as I was, but what can you do? Why is it important to practice self-care? The quality of life of every nurse and the existence of the nursing profession greatly depend on self-care being implemented in the lives of every healthcare professional Nurses are good at providing quality care and direction to others, but when it comes to abiding by that same personal guidance and instructions, we are not as good. Health promotion models have taught us that people change when there is a significant reason to change. When I have the threat of a cavity, I can floss daily. When a woman learns she is pregnant, she can put down cigarettes. People often can change their eating habits when given a choice of diet modification or medication for a lifetime. What will be the motivating factor for nurses to determine that self-care is not an option? There are many nurses who are leading full, satisfying lives. Self-care is still needed. There are many nurses who are not leading the full, satisfying lives that they wish they could. Self-care is still needed. Self-care is for prevention, self-care is for maintenance, and self-care is for damage control. Self-care is about being educated before we reach the levels where damage control is needed; however, it is always there when we need it. Often we are so busy meeting the needs of others, we may fail to realize what we need ourselves. I didn't know I was experiencing burnout after being a nurse for only a few years, but I knew that the person I was on the inside was not who I was displaying on the outside. I couldn't figure out why.

Determining Your Self-Care Group

There are three categories of nurses who engage in self-care at some point in their careers. The first group consists of nurses who practice self-care on a daily basis and are enjoying satisfaction in many areas of life. The second group includes nurses who do not practice self-care or practice it so infrequently that they don't know they are doing so, and are not consistently enjoying satisfaction in various areas of life. The third group includes nurses who practice self-care inconsistently and thus experience inconsistent benefits. The key is to keep the first group engaged in the ongoing practice of self-care, because they are a definite strength in health care and the work environment and a beacon of light to nurses who cross their paths. The key for the second and third groups is to provide adequate education on self-care, including its benefits and how it impacts our lifestyles and careers. This is a seed-planting stage that allows us to introduce concepts that many nurses may not be totally familiar with, relating to what self-care truly is. For those of you who are finding your way, determine where you are currently and accept yourself for where you are. In time you will be able to advance yourself to a stage of change by practicing the exercises and having will and determination.

The self-care exercises in this chapter are fun and simple. They are called "setting the intention" and "creating a sacred space." These two exercises will help you set the pace for the rest of your reading journey.

BEGINNING YOUR JOURNEY

Setting the Intention

I find it so amazing to watch babies as they learn to crawl and begin to explore the power of mobility. I can recall my own children in those stages, patiently and diligently scooting their little bodies across the floor to obtain an object of interest on the other side of the room (like our beautifully lit and attractive Christmas Tree!). Intention begins with a thought to achieve, coupled with the persistence to make that achievement manifest. Within this equation of thought and persistence is the power of the intention. The concept of intention is addressed in more detail in another chapter. Here, let's simply think about what we desire to accomplish from reading this book. Perhaps we want to support holistic beliefs we may already have, or learn more about holistic therapies, how to take better care of ourselves and coworkers, or how to manage our staff in holistic and nurturing ways. Whatever the case may be, now is the perfect time for you to sit with your thoughts and imagine what this journey will look, taste, feel, and sound like. My personal intention in writing this book is to help facilitate a transformation in the consciousness of members of the nursing profession so that they will see the necessity of incorporating self-care, compassion, and nurturing in their daily lives, as well as the lives of their colleagues, to maintain a healthy balance.

There is another meaning for the word "intention," and it is used in relation to our awareness of the healing potential for others, on levels that we are not in control of, responsible for, or attached to. This definition of intention is "the conscious awareness of being in the present moment to help facilitate the healing process; a volitional act of love" (Dossey & Keegan, 2009, p. 49). Take a moment to sit with this definition and experience how it feels and sounds to you as well. You have the freedom and permission to make your own personal healing and commitment to self-love an intention for reading this book. There is no right or wrong way to set your intentions. The key to begin exploring what you can create for yourself is to see it within your mind's eye! Table 1-3 illustrates an example of setting your intentions, and Table 1-4 illustrates an example of your intentions for reading this book.

Creating a Sacred Space

Having first set our intentions, we are well on our way to setting the holistic mood for our book-reading pleasure. Although setting the intention and creating a sacred space are not requirements, they can be very beneficial to you. Both activities help you to shift toward moving toward a higher consciousness. By setting your intention, you can discover your mind's power to create your reality, and by creating a sacred space you can create a conscious place in which to meet your needs for relaxation, discovery, self-care, and so much more. You

---

Table 1-3   Example of Setting Intentions

> I, Rachel Y. Hill, on the 20th day of January,
> set forth my intention for writing "Nursing from the Inside-Out".
>
> My intention for writing the book "Nursing from the Inside-Out" is to help facilitate a transformation in the consciousness of the nursing profession so that we find it pertinent to incorporate self-care, compassion, and nurturance for ourselves, in every action, so that we are able to equally care for others and maintain balance in our daily lives.
>
> This/these intention(s) is/are based on what I know to feel right within my heart and to be true for myself. It is my responsibility to support my intentions with action, patience, and diligence; while keeping an open mind to the many possibilities available (seen and unseen) for fulfilling my intention(s), beyond my wildest dreams! I have total trust in the guidance of my inner wisdom. It is done!
>
> Rachel Y. Hill, ARNP, FNP-BC

Table 1-4   My Intentions

I, _____, on the ____ day of _____,
set forth my intention for reading "Nursing from the Inside-Out".

My intention(s) is/are

_____

_____

_____

_____

This/these intention(s) is/are based on what I know to feel right within my heart and to be true for myself. It is my responsibility to support my intentions with action, patience, and diligence; while keeping an open mind to the many possibilities available (seen and unseen) for fulfilling my intention(s), beyond my wildest dreams! I have total trust in the guidance of my inner wisdom. It is done!

_____

Your signature

---

have started the process of joining your subconscious mind and conscious mind together to begin this wonderful journey. Finding a space that you have created and are willing to dedicate to your own personal self-care rituals sends a very strong message to yourself. The message serves to strengthen your mind's perception of the commitment you have made to fulfill your intentions and to be true to yourself (as an individual and as a nursing professional). I don't doubt that some of you might feel that the act of creating a sacred space and enjoying it is practically impossible, especially if you have a large patient load and a few new admits sprinkled on top. I remember (as I'm sure many of you do) the days when I had a house full of small children. I thought it would be many decades before I could ever use the restroom alone and uninterrupted. Creating a sacred space definitely did not seem like a viable concept for me at that time. However, if you have a desire to step out of the rat race, make the effort. Even if the effort is a little one, it will go a long way. Luke (17:6) says basically that if you have the faith of a mustard seed, you can move mountains, and change is only challenging when you struggle against it. What I also now realize is that the physical "sacred space" we are making the effort to create will ultimately become a state of mind that will exist with every thought and action. This special place within is our place of peace and inner sanctuary. When the call lights are going off, patients are severely restless, and the nursing shortage is directly impacting you, but you can still feel that total peace within yourself, you will have achieved the ultimate goal of creating a sacred space. Regardless of where we go, the "peace within" will always be present and accessible to us. How to make this within-space accessible is definitely up to us, because we will have all the tools necessary to explore it. In the meantime, we will put our energy and loving thoughts toward creating an external sacred space. This space can be set up in a special corner, room, closet, attic, or wherever you are able to find space to honor yourself. I cleared out my dining room (because our food never seemed to make it past the kitchen anyway) and set up my special sacred space to be alone and revive myself every day.

1. Select the area in which you will create a sacred space for yourself or your group. Suggestions: a corner, room, closet, break room, spare office, attic, basement, etc.

2. Clean and sanitize your space accordingly. If your sacred space is in the attic, you might need to box with the dust bunnies a little. Be kind to yourself and your environment in doing so. Air purifiers are great too! If you are sharing space with others, be sure to make it a group effort. If you have windows that can be opened, and the availability of sunshine, consider yourself very lucky and use them for the good of your space. Sunshine is healing and fresh air is so invigorating. There are many ways to clean your space spiritually as well. You can take clary sage (purchased from herbal shops, Whole Foods, New Age bookstores, etc.), light it, and walk around your space with the smoke from the sage smoldering. You can take the sage smoke and act as if you are dusting your space with it. "Dust" the corners of the room, the walls, the ceiling, the floor, and all of the objects that are in your space.

3. Add your individual and/or group's personal touches to the room. This fills the room up with the positive energy of the individual or group. The personal touches should reflect one's intentions, and can be things that are reverenced and held dear, symbols of people who are inspiring, or objects that are soothing to the eye and healing to the spirit. Special music, pictures, plants, blankets, bells and chimes, fountains, artwork, candles, throw rugs, and nice pillows to sit on are just a few things that are personal and enhance your sacred space. You want a place that is kind and comforting to you. A word of caution to individuals and groups: avoid cluttering your space. If you feel you have too much to put in your room, and don't have a stopping mechanism within yourself, remember that when you do your regular cleanup (biweekly or monthly), you can remodel your space so that

you will always have a new look and freshness! Try to include symbols that express your thoughts, define who you are, and express what you desire in your life, specifically I have a massage table in my room, which I find very useful. Whenever my children are not feeling well, I give them liberty to go into my room and rest. They always migrate to that table when they are feeling out of harmony and in need of a little pick-me-up.

4. Once your space is completed to your liking and specifications, you can honor it in a way that is special for you. You may want to have a candle-lighting ceremony in which you light a candle and say a prayer. You may want to burn incense, sing a song, or say a prayer to welcome love and light within your space. Rituals are not necessary, but often such actions can help enhance the already existing miracles we create in our daily lives through faith and believing.

5. Enjoy your space and visit it frequently. Create a brain pathway that associates that room with your need to heal and rejuvenate. At the end of your workday, after you have cleaned up, go to your room and meditate, pray, or listen to relaxing music. It's as simple as that. You create a pattern of nurturing and replenishing yourself. Enjoy!

REFERENCES

Andrus, V. (2005). Caring for self: Becoming a healing presence. *AHNA Beginnings, 1,* 20.

Donley, S. R. (2005). Challenges for nursing in the 21st century. *Nursing Economics, 23* (6), 312–318.

Dossey, B. M., & Keegan, L. (2009). *Holistic nursing: A handbook for practice.* Sudbury, MA: Jones and Bartlett.

Koopsen, C., & Young, C. (2009). *Integrative health: A holistic approach for health professionals.* Sudbury, MA: Jones and Bartlett.

Van Wagner, K. (n.d.). *Hierarchy of Needs: The Five Levels of Maslow's Hierarchy of Needs.* Retrieved June 24, 2009, from www.About.com: http://psychology.about.com/od/theoriesofpersonality/a/hierarchyneeds.htm?p=1

SUGGESTED READING LIST

Anonymous. (2007). Investing in nursing's future: PIN projects in Montana, Mississippi, Michigan and six other states. *Nursing Education Perspectives, 28,* 242–243.

Buerhaus, P. I., Donelan, K., Ulrich, B. T., Norman, L., DesRoches, C., & Dittus, R. (2007). Impact of the nurse shortage on hospital patient care: Comparative perspectives. *Health Affairs, 26,* 853–862.

Bush, N. J. (2009). Compassion fatigue: Are you at risk? *Oncology Nursing Forum, 36,* 24–28.

Donley, S. R. (2005). Challenges for nursing in the 21st century. *Nursing Economics, 23*(6), 312–318.

Letvak, S., & Buck, R. (2008). Factors influencing work productivity and intent to stay in nursing. *Nurse Economy, 26*(3), 159–165.

Lutz, S. L., & Root, D. (2007). Nurses, consumer satisfaction, and pay for performance. *Healthcare Financial Management, 61,* 57–63.

Shirey, M. (2006). Stress and coping in nurse managers: Two decades of research. *Nurse Economics, 24*(4), 193–203, 211.

CHAPTER 2

Introduction to Jin Shin Jyutsu®
Physio-Philosophy

RACHEL Y. HILL

"Seek that which has no beginning or ending,
but the journey that lies within."

—MARY BURMEISTER

INTRODUCTION TO JIN SHIN JYUTSU® PHYSIO-PHILOSOPHY

The body shivers when it is cold, in an effort to automatically warm itself. A scab forms within minutes of a cut, in an effort to stop bleeding. The eyes blink instantly, in an effort to protect themselves from foreign objects. These are automatic functions of the body that under normal circumstances tend to themselves. The human body is a fascinating creation, unlike any other. Psalms 139:14 in the Bible says, "I will praise thee; for I am fearfully and wonderfully made: marvelous are thy works; and that my soul knoweth right well." The body has the innate ability to heal itself. This was something we knew very well once upon a time. We have since forgotten our abilities, but every day, these forgotten abilities resurface without our ever knowing what we are attempting to do. What happens when we forget our car keys or our name badge? We might first blame it on a "senior moment." However, in the world of Jin Shin Jyutsu, that type of moment doesn't exist. There is an imbalance occurring that requires a shift. We stop, place our hands on top of our heads, and begin to think about where the missing item could be. Instantly, a mental image or the thought of a location leads us to where it is. We have just tapped into the forgotten mystery of energy and performed a little Jin Shin Jyutsu on ourselves. Think about those extended nursing lectures, meetings on policies and procedures, etc., that you have to attend. Sometimes you don't quite know whether you will make it through. You are either tired or ready to fall asleep, or you are freezing because the room is too cold. You sit on your hands, applying a comfortable pressure as they rest securely underneath your bottom. The energy begins to return to your body and you begin to feel restored. Your temperature begins to rise and become regulated, and you begin to feel like you could sit through 6 more hours of the lecture. You are again subconsciously experiencing the power of Jin Shin Jyutsu within yourself.

These are things that we were once conscious of but have been lost to us over time. Fortunately, the healing practice is reemerging and we are able to reawaken and recapture many things that our consciousness has forgotten.

History of Jin Shin Jyutsu

Learning the history of Jin Shin Jyutsu is one of the favorite parts of my experience. In my personal experience of taking the courses, the history of Jin Shin Jyutsu has never been told to me the same way twice. The basis is pretty much the same each time, though, with a little bit of the storyteller's personality thrown into it. I have had many teachers, who each shared what he or she had been told. I enjoyed each version as if I was hearing it for the first time. Some of what I heard was history, and some of what I heard was mystery; however, the details do not concern me much. The important things are the art form itself and the concepts that are being shared with others and utilized daily. One of the beauties of this ancient healing tradition is that it has been passed down for thousands of years by word of mouth. I am connected to the Jin Shin Jyutsu legacy. In keeping with the ancient traditions, I want to share this legacy as accurately as I know how, and I am honored to pass the story on to you. I encourage you to study thoroughly and experience the history in your own way, just as I have experienced it in mine, and continue to pass it on.

Jin means man of knowing, compassion. *Shin* means universal intelligence or life force, spirit, or creator. *Jyutsu* means the self. Thus, the combined meaning of Jin Shin Jyutsu is the art of knowing oneself. Jin Shin Jyutsu is an ancient form of healing whose roots extend deep into the times of Moses and Gautama Buddha more than 3000 years ago. Jin Shin Jyutsu was reintroduced to Japan in the early 1900s by way of Master Jiro Murai. In the 1950s, Jin Shin Jyutsu was introduced in the United States by way of Mary Burmeister, a student of Master Jiro Murai. This healing art form had been forgotten for thousands of years, and there was little written documentation because the ancient healing practices had been passed down verbally from one generation to the next. Since its rediscovery, we have been able to create more documentation on Jin Shin Jyutsu; however, there are still thousands of years unaccounted for. There is only one remaining document that contains any written information regarding Jin Shin Jyutsu. This collection of writings is called the Kojiki, or the Japanese Record of Ancient Things. These writings date back to 712 A.D. The Kojiki is a collection of many stories about the creation of the world and the battles, lives, and relationships of gods and goddesses. I have not personally read the Kojiki, but it is said to carry symbols that contain healing messages within the writing.

Master Jiro Murai

Master Jiro Murai was born into a family of medical physicians. In Japanese tradition, it is customary for the eldest to take up the profession of the father.

Master Jiro's older brothers became physicians like their father. Master Jiro was the younger of his brothers and did not have the pressure of tradition. He pursued a career as a silkworm herder instead of being a doctor. Master Jiro Murai had also been known to indulge in eating and drinking contests in his youth, which led to a severe illness. The illness he suffered was incurable. Jiro Murai became so ill that he made a conscious decision to separate himself from his family, whom he had disgraced, and let his fate run its course. His family took him to their cabin in the mountains to be left alone for 7 days. They were instructed to return on the eighth day. His family did not expect to see him alive again.

During Jiro Murai's time alone, he meditated on all the teachings of the masters he had learned through oral tradition. He began to practice all of what he could remember about the forgotten art of Jin Shin Jyutsu on himself. Daily, his body temperature dropped as he moved in and out of consciousness. On the seventh day, he suddenly felt himself being lifted out of his semi-frozen state and exposed to an extreme amount of heat like a furnace. When his fever subsided, his consciousness returned and he felt completely well and healed. He was so grateful that he fell to his knees and gave thanks to his Creator, and made a personal vow that he would spend the rest of his life researching this wonderful art. When his family returned, he was sitting out in front of the cabin (maybe on the porch, maybe on a big rock or a tree stump). I can imagine a big grin on his face when he saw the confused expressions on the faces of his family as they returned to carry his body away.

Master Jiro Murai kept true to his word and began to document all the things he had experienced and rediscovered on the mountain. Once he had gathered all his information, he took it to the library so that the results of his research could be kept in the records of his country. However, the librarian told him that his information was a duplicate. They already had information in their records very similar to what he had submitted to them. The librarian presented him with the Kojiki, and Master Jiro Murai realized that this information had been around all the time. Jin Shin Jyutsu had just been reawakened by his experience. As it says in the Bible, "What has been is what will be, and what has been done is what will be done; and there is nothing new under the sun" (Ecclesiastes 1:9).

Mary Burmeister

In the 1940s, Mary Burmeister met Master Jiro Murai. She was a first-generation Japanese American born in Seattle, Washington. It was said that Mary went to Japan to learn the Japanese language. She had absolutely no clue what life held in store for her on this journey. While in Japan, she was asked to tutor a woman in English. She became sick and was ill enough to require medical attention.

Through the illness she experienced, she met Master Jiro Murai. The first words he ever spoke to her were, "How would you like to study with me and take a gift from Japan to America?" In other versions of the story, Mary met Master Jiro Murai before she grew gravely ill. Master Jiro Murai's dedication to helping her and sharing the art of healing was enough to convince her of the higher meaning that Jin Shin Jyutsu would have in her life. Mary had never been sick and took it for granted that people who were sick were trying to find ways to avoid their responsibilities in life. Experiencing a severe illness herself gave her an opportunity to experience the path of those she would help, and put her in a better position to help others who were in need. "Afterward, she understood that suffering is not feigned. This realization infused her with the compassion necessary to pursue a life devoted to helping others" (Burmeister & Monte, 1997).

Dr. Haruki Kato

During this same time, a Japanese medical physician, Dr. Haruki Kato, was offered the same opportunity as Mary to study with Master Jiro Murai. From what I gathered, he has been able to apply Jin Shin Jyutsu from a different perspective, and still teaches the art today to medical professionals in Japan. I have heard that he has lectured in the United States and shared his teachings based on what he learned from Master Jiro Murai.

Mary studied with Master Jiro Murai for 5 years in Japan, and continued to correspond with him for about 7 more years after she returned to the United States. As the story goes, it was about 17 more years before Mary Burmeister felt comfortable enough to begin sharing the art of Jin Shin Jyutsu with others. She finally realized that with such an art form, you will never stop learning. She began working with various people and the word spread, which increased her confidence and her opportunities to share Jin Shin Jyutsu with others. According to my teachers, Mary's living room was often filled with kids from her children's school, who were receiving Jin Shin Jyutsu for healing.

Mary began to document and draw the things that she had been taught by Master Jiro Murai, and to formalize the teachings that she would introduce to the world and share with healthcare professionals from many different countries. Jin Shin Jyutsu is taught globally, in several languages, and used for both humans and animals. Master Jiro Murai's intuition to share Jin Shin Jyutsu with Mary has impacted the movement of energy healing in the healthcare setting. When the student is ready, the teacher appears. His teachings were well received by Mary and dispersed to the world, beyond what Master Jiro imagined (or maybe exactly how he imagined).

Mary Burmeister transitioned from this life on January 27, 2008. Her family continues to live out the legacy she left behind, to keep the art form of Jin

Shin Jyutsu and its mission alive. The Jin Shin Jyutsu mission statement is as follows:

> Through the dynamic Art of Jin Shin Jyutsu (Physio-Philosophy), our mission IS to create a safe environment for reawakening the true SELF. Being the testimony of this simple, profound Art of Living, made known to us by Mary Burmeister and Jiro Murai, we educate, harmonize and inspire ourselves and others through integrity, compassion, trust and freedom to BE...NOW KNOW MYSELF.

Concepts of Jin Shin Jyutsu

Jin Shin Jyutsu is not a technique or a modality. Jin Shin Jyutsu is an art form. The Merriam-Webster online dictionary (2009) defines art as "the conscious use of skill and creative imagination, especially in the production of aesthetic objects." Once we begin to study and apply Jin Shin Jyutsu, we begin to learn that we are born with an innate ability to heal ourselves. By experiencing Jin Shin Jyutsu, we begin to gather the knowledge to fulfill that healing potential. The creativity of that information is expressed in our beautifully designed bodies through health, wellness, and self-awareness.

Jin Shin Jyutsu is Japanese acupressure. This art form uses the simple touch of the hands and the "breath" to balance the life force within the body. The breath can be described as an expression of the life force energy. Every living being is full of this energy or life force. "The ancient Greeks referred to this energy as pneuma; the Hindus call it prana; the Chinese know it as chi (also qi), and the Japanese, ki" (Burmeister & Monte, 1997). Another concept is that the universal life force energy manifests itself in different levels in our being, called depths. Each breath we inhale, we receive the essence of our existence, and with each exhale we are able to release blocked energy and cleanse the unnecessary accumulations within us. When we don't release these accumulations, we experience illness, disease, and pain (mental, spiritual, or physical).

In Jin Shin Jyutsu, illness and disease are called labels or disharmonies. Headaches are considered labels. Cancer is a label. Heartburn is label. Some labels are more serious than others, but all are blockages that prevent the life force energy from flowing freely. Another concept is that energy is constantly moving in an oval down the front and up the back of our bodies. This movement is creating a connection between the back and front of the body, and the upper and lower halves of the body. We are able to look to the lower half when we are experiencing disharmony in the upper half of the body, and vice versa.

The blockages that are created in our bodies are created by attitudes we possess at different times that are not in harmony with who we truly are. Those attitudes are worry, fear, anger, anxiety, grief, and pretense. When we dwell in unhealthy attitudes for long periods of time, it creates an opportunity for blocked energy to accumulate. Jin Shin Jyutsu is used to move the blocked energy so that balance of the life force can be restored. The body is made up of 26 safety energy locks. These safety energy locks are arranged in pairs that serve as circuit breakers in the body. Draw a vertical line down the center of your body. You have 26 safety energy locks on the right side of the vertical line and 26 safety energy locks that are mirrored on the left side. When the electrical circuits in our homes experience a power surge, the circuit breaker flips off to protect the system. The safety energy locks work the same way. They shut off to protect the body and warn us that something is going on that needs our immediate attention (such as trauma, exposure to viruses, toxins, or bacteria, etc.). Once we are alerted, we can give our attention to relieving these blockages by creating various flows or patterns in which we move energy through the body by using our hands.

With the simple application of the hands to certain parts of an individual's body, one can help move energy and establish balance to the body. The skilled practitioner carries out an assessment that entails listening to the body's pulse by feeling it in the wrists, so that he or she can know which flow will be useful in removing the blockage. The imbalance is detected in the pulse of the individual. The practitioner serves as "jumper cable," recharging the life force within the person being treated. The pulses felt in the wrist differ from the radial pulse we use to measure the heart rate of a patient. These pulses are felt two times in each wrist. The first pulse is taken with three fingers on a superficial level (lightly touching the inner wrist with the fingers). The second pulse is taken on a deeper level, with the fingers pressing more into the wrist. Each pulse provides very helpful information because it helps indicate where the blockages are and what types of flows are needed to help the individual. For treatment, a grounding hand is kept on the body at all times, and a floating hand is moved to different parts of the body during the balancing. When the pulses felt by the grounding hand and the floating hand beat as one, synchrony is established. The practitioner can then move to the next place in the flow pattern, until the flow is complete.

Jin Shin Jyutsu is not massage. When people hear the word "acupressure," they seem to automatically think of needles. However, there are no needles involved in the practice of Jin Shin Jyutsu. There are no physical manipulations of any kind. The effects of Jin Shin Jyutsu are able to penetrate skin, clothing, and cast-like materials. You can do no harm when performing Jin Shin Jyutsu on yourself or on others. All that is required of you is the intention to help others for the highest good. Mary Burmeister would often tell others that we cannot make mistakes when sharing Jin Shin Jyutsu, because we are only helping to harmonize the body with our hands. Jin Shin Jyutsu does not replace the medical treatment of a health practitioner and is not associated with a religion of any sort. However, it complements conventional medicine as well as religious beliefs.

Terms Related to Jin Shin Jyutsu

The following terms may be unfamiliar to you but are commonly used when discussing concepts related to Jin Shin Jyutsu:

Attitudes – Obstructions in the free flow of the life force energy that can lead to physical, mental, and emotional imbalances.

Breath – It is through the breath that the life force is shown and expressed.

Depths – The life force energy is expressed at different levels of density.

Disease – Disharmony in the body; blocked or stagnated energy.

Energy – The life force that flows through the body.

Energy pathways – The life force energy that goes down the front of the body and up the back, along the 12 organ flows.

Flows – Specific pathways in which the life force energy travels through the body.

Harmony – The state in which the life force energy is able to flow freely.

Jumper cabling – Applying the life force energy throughout the body, using one's hands. One hand is kept grounded on the body while the other hand moves to different parts of the body. The energy penetrates clothing, casts, shoes, or braces.

Labels – The disharmonies we experience, such as HIV, cancer, and diabetes. The labels can be big or small.

Life force – An energy that dwells within all living creatures.

Project – A proactive and positive word that allows us to look at issues and situations as being solvable. Any issue we face is the work of our lives in progress. Projects are experiences that require planning and objectivity, so that we can execute our plans and learn from the project itself. A term that has traditionally been used is "problem." Problems tend to have a negative undertone, with little vibration of hope and victory in overcoming them.

Safety energy locks – The body has 26 special places, identical on each side of the body, that are used to protect the body when it is in disharmony. They are often compared to circuit breakers. When there is a surge, the circuit switches off to protect the source. When energy is blocked in the body, the safety energy lock develops a symptom that alerts us to the presence of disharmony.

Self-Care Practices (Also Referred to as Jin Shin Jyutsu Self-Help)

Self-care is so important in Jin Shin Jyutsu that there are three books dedicated to its daily practice. There are three ways to experience the art of Jin Shin Jyutsu for yourself: (1) You can receive treatments from a certified Jin Shin Jyutsu practitioner, (2) you can learn self-help practices and use them daily, and/or (3) you can seek out self-help groups in your area and receive treatments from others (while learning more about Jin Shin Jyutsu). Jin Shin Jyutsu is great to experience through practitioners, because you can allow yourself to be in a mode of receiving. Self-care doesn't get any better than that. It is a nice treat to give yourself at the end of a busy workday or hectic week, or just for the health and well-being of your body. During the first or second visit with a practitioner, he or she will begin teaching you different self-help tools for daily maintenance. Practicing daily self-maintenance, self-help, or self-care is how one learns to "know oneself" through Jin Shin Jyutsu.

A practitioner won't always be available 24/7 when a *now* need arises. Jin Shin Jyutsu does not replace regular or acute medical treatment—it serves as a complement to other therapies. Jin Shin Jyutsu encourages self-sufficiency and empowers you to rely on your innate ability to heal yourself. This is the second way to experience Jin Shin Jyutsu through self-help. Have you ever heard the ancient proverb, "Give a man a fish, you will feed him for a day; teach a man to fish, and you will feed him for a lifetime"? Once you have established a self-help routine, you will develop a sense of self-reliance. The self-reliance fosters well-being. The well-being fosters knowing. Thus, your ability to hear and understand what your body is saying (through the signals that the safety energy locks give off) increases. The "self-help flows" described later in this chapter are just a sample of the endless possibilities that can be a part of everyday experience. There is so much power in a simple touch. Jin Shin Jyutsu is about doing and not trying. So of course, through daily practice, you get to experience who you really are.

Like nurses, practitioners are caregivers. In Jin Shin Jyutsu seminars, practitioners are highly encouraged to practice self-help every day to keep themselves balanced and healthy. Jin Shin Jyutsu does not weaken a practitioner, because the practitioner is only helping to facilitate the movement of energy throughout the body. However, the practitioner is a human being who has the potential to become imbalanced. The self-help tools are used for maintenance, and enable the practitioner to get out of his or her "pickle" much faster by simply applying the self-help practices that are utilized in Jin Shin Jyutsu. If you don't have a Jin Shin Jyutsu practitioner, you can officially be your own practitioner.

There are number of "self-help practices" (beyond what has been included in this section) that are equal to the term "self-care" in Jin Shin Jyutsu. You are invited to spend time experiencing each self-help practice in whatever order you choose. You can study one self-help practice each day, each week, or even each month to become familiar with its benefits and how it impacts your health and well-being at home and at work. There is no right or wrong way to practice Jin Shin Jyutsu self-help, and the good news is that you have the tools (your hands and your breath) with you no matter where you go. The key is that you practice self-help exercises and explore. Decide which course you wish to take and begin the journey. You may find it helpful to keep a journal of your experiences, reflecting on what flows have been useful to you, how they have affected your outcomes for the day, and what you have learned from each experience. Use Jin Shin Jyutsu at home for yourself. Once you have established your own self-help routine and are familiar with the practices, feel free to pass the information and benefits on to others. The same scenario applies to work. Once you have experienced the different self-help flows offered, you can begin to share self-help with coworkers, patients, and others who may need to learn how to care for themselves more deeply.

During this time, treat yourself with the most loving care that you would extend to a patient, client, family member, or friend. Take this opportunity to honor yourself by becoming aware of your body's energy flow, identifying any blockages you may have, and working toward releasing the stagnation. You are still learning, so be kind and gentle to yourself. You are fishing for a lifetime!

Main Central Flow

Description:

The Main Central Flow (Fig. 2-1) is a centering flow that serves to tune and harmonize the body. "This is our Source of Life. We are as harmonious or out of rhythm as is the energy supply from this source. In fact, this is our present state

Figure 2-1   Main central flow.

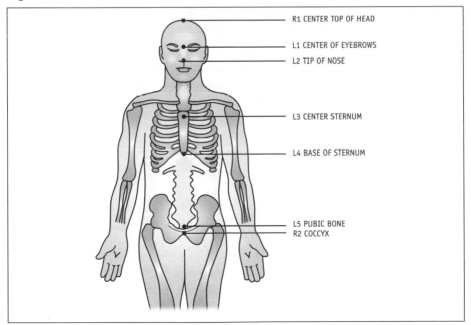

R1 CENTER TOP OF HEAD

L1 CENTER OF EYEBROWS

L2 TIP OF NOSE

L3 CENTER STERNUM

L4 BASE OF STERNUM

L5 PUBIC BONE
R2 COCCYX

of being-in health or ailing" (Burmeister, 1994). The practitioner applies light pressure with each step. The hand placements for the main central vertical flow are on the spinal column, including the seven major chakras (later we discuss how many ancient healing forms are connected and similar to one another in this regard). The effects of the flow are very calming and relaxing, and only require you to relax and breath. The Main Central Flow serves to provide what is needed for that time. If energy is needed for the body, the Main Central Flow will energize. If relaxation is needed, the Main Central Flow will help the body achieve relaxation. It is all based on balancing your needs.

Find a cozy place to sit or lie down. If you have created a sacred space, as discussed in the beginning of this book, you can go there. Review the diagram and the positions; most importantly, relax. Follow the hand positions and keep things simple. There is no way to perform the Main Central Flow incorrectly. Your hands end up where they end up, because that is simply what you require for that moment. Set your intention to be open and receive from the experience. Be aware of your thoughts and feelings before, during, and after this experience. Honor who you are and how you are feeling. As mentioned earlier, you may want to practice this flow for a longer period of time, say a week, a month, or even 90 days. After the exercise and each time you do the Main Central Flow, ground yourself by taking in deep breaths, wiggle and shake your hands and feet, and take some time to record your feelings in your journal.

This flow can be done during any time of the day, but I prefer to do it in the morning upon rising and at night before going to bed. This following diagram illustrates the main central vertical flow and is a simple tool that I use quite frequently to regain balance. The right hand rests on the center top of the head. The left hand moves down the body to each of five positions (the center of the eyebrows, tip of the nose, center of the sternum, base of the sternum, and pubic bone). In each position, the hands are held briefly for 1 to 2 minutes, or until a gentle pulsation is noted. In the final step, the right hand moves down to the coccyx.

The Steps:

1. Place the fingers of your right hand on top of your head (where they will remain until step 6).
2. Place the fingers of your left hand on your forehead between your eyebrows. Hold for 3 to 5 minutes or until the pulses you feel at your fingertips beat as one with each other.
3. Move your left fingertips to the tip of your nose. Hold them there for 3 to 5 minutes, or until the pulses beat as one with each other.
4. Move your left fingertips to your sternum (the center of your chest between your breasts). Stay there for 3 to 5 minutes, or until the pulses beat in sync with each other.

5. Move your left fingertips to the base of your sternum. Hold them there for 3 to 5 minutes, or until the pulses beat in sync with each other.
6. Move the fingers of your left hand to the top of your pubis. Stay there for 3 to 5 minutes, or until the pulses beat in sync with each other.
7. Keep your left fingertips in place while you move your right fingertips to cover your coccyx. Hold this place for 3 to 5 minutes or until the pulses you feel at your fingertips beat in sync with each other.
8. If you are recording your experiences, be sure to take note of how you feel before and after the exercise. If you are reading this book as part of a group, share your experience with others, if you feel comfortable doing so.
9. As the final step, move your right hand from the top of your head to your coccyx.

Benefits of self-care:

- Helps us maintain the life force energy in intense situations.
- Grounds us for the upcoming day.
- Balances and calms the body after stressful or traumatic experiences.
- Provides relaxation and stress relief before, during, and after work.
- Provides relaxation and stress relief at home.
- Centers and clears the mind so that one can act quickly when needed.
- Energizes the body when one is tired, or relaxes the body when one is hyper.

36 Breaths

Description:

Everywhere we go, so goes our breath. This is one tool that is at our disposal whenever we need it. In times of stress or emergency, all we have to remember is to slow our breathing down, relax our shoulders, and take in the opportunity for learning at that moment. This is one of the most important tools we have to heal ourselves. As we inhale and exhale consciously, we are able to experience a deeper connection with our life force energy. When we take our time to inhale and savor each breath slowly and consciously, we receive the life force energy that is abundant and available for us all. This life force energy connects our body, mind, and spirit. When we consciously exhale and release, we let go of stressors and tension that cause accumulations within us.

The Steps:

Find a comfortable place. You can be sitting up with your spine straight or resting flat on your back. Do not practice this breathing exercise while driving. To perform the 36 Breaths exercise, you exhale and then inhale in a relaxed manner. Each cycle of exhalation/inhalation counts as one breath. Therefore, all you have to do is count each exhalation until it has been done 36 times. (If you lose your place during your breathing, simply start over again.) Once more, if you are keeping a journal, take note of how you feel before and after the exercise. Write your feelings down and honor who you are. If you are reading this book as part of a group, share your experience with others, if you feel comfortable doing so.

Benefits of self-care:

- Provides clarity and peace of mind.
- Oxygenates the cells.
- Helps cleanse the body.
- Improves and produces relaxation.
- Increases mood elevation.
- Helps improve sleeping.

The Attitudes

Description:

A few years ago, a very popular expression was "Talk to the hand!" This phrase was generally used when someone no longer wanted to listen to what another person was saying. Jin Shin Jyutsu encourages the practice of "talking to the hand," in a much kinder and more compassionate way. The hand represents attitudes (illustrated in Fig. 2-2) that lead to imbalances in our bodies. If you're experiencing worry, talk to the hand! If you're experiencing fear, talk to the hand! If you're experiencing any of the attitudes that can cause blockages in your body, talk to the hand! By communicating with our hands, we can achieve the balance that we are in need of. The hand (fingers and palms) is a simple and potent self-help tool to harmonize and bring the body into balance. Each finger of the hand represents an attitude we possess in our daily life. The attitudes are the main contributors to our energy becoming blocked and stagnant within our bodies. In Jin Shin Jyutsu, we use the expression "Rid (palms) Worry (thumbs) FAST" (F stands for fear and relates to the index finger, A stands for anger and relates to the middle finger, S stands for sadness and relates to the ring finger, and T stands for trying too hard and relates to the pinky).

The palm of the hand represents clearing out the attitudes quickly (Rid Worry FAST). If we can keep our attitudes in check, we can go with the flow (literally) and live more harmonized lives.

You can experience this exercise in a nice quiet setting initially, but realistically, you will probably need to do this exercise in many places. That means you may not always have peace and/or quiet. You could be anywhere when you need to bring yourself into balance, so remember you have everything you need with you at all times. Described below are two ways to bring yourself into balance.

Figure 2-2   The attitudes.

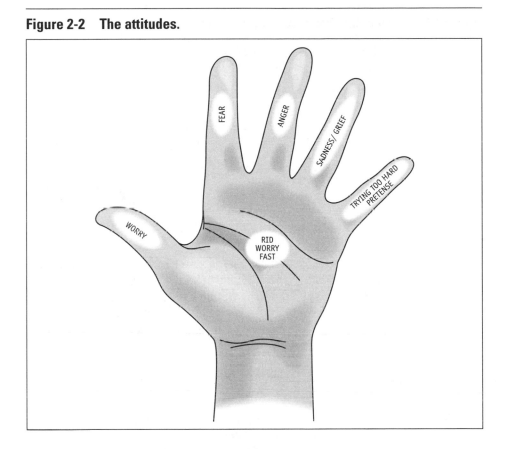

The first method is the "quickie" method, for when you're really pushed for time or need to achieve balance in a hurry. The second is a longer sequence that is included for your self-care. Try one or try them both.

When you are experiencing an attitude, simply hold the finger of the attitude you are experiencing at that time and breathe. This helps release tension and stress.

Description: Thumb

The thumb represents worry. The television series "Happy Days" featured a motorcycle-riding heartthrob, Arthur Fonzarelli ("the Fonz"). He would always give a thumbs-up and say "AAAAAY!" to signify that everything was "cool," or, in other words, there was nothing to worry about. Babies can't communicate with us about their imbalances, but they will often suck their thumbs to help establish a balance within themselves.

Figure 2-3   The quickie thumb-worry (left hand).

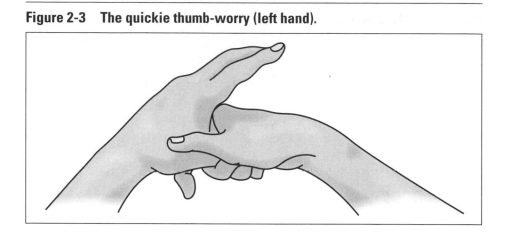

For this exercise, simply wrap your hand around your left thumb and hold it there for a few minutes (Fig. 2-3), then wrap your hand around your right thumb and hold it for a few minutes (Fig. 2-4). Holding the thumb supports the following issues: depression, hate, obsession, anxiety, self-protection, physical fatigue, problems in the back of the head, breathing, and digestive discomforts (Burmeister, 1994).

Benefits of self-care:

- Alleviates difficulty sleeping.
- Improves digestion.
- Supports back weakness.
- Helps alleviate skin rashes and blemishes.
- Supports issues in prosperity and abundance or financial well-being.

Figure 2-4   The quickie thumb – worry (right hand).

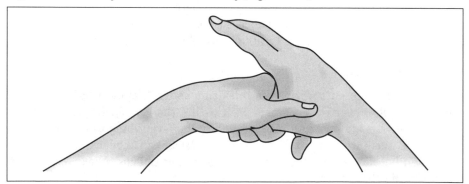

Figure 2-5   The quickie index finger-fear (left hand).

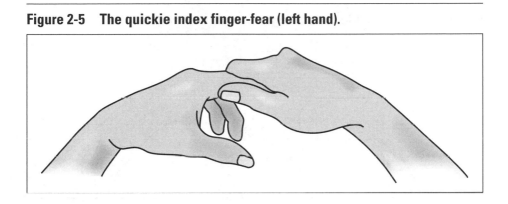

- Alleviates weight imbalances.
- Comforts the worrywart.

Description: Index finger

The index finger represents fear. When we point at others in blame, we have four fingers pointing right back at us. The picture of Uncle Sam shows a man dressed in red, white, and blue pointing out to "YOU," encouraging you to join the military and fight for our country. Uncle Sam is pretty famous, but he was probably too busy pointing to join the military himself. For this exercise, simply wrap your hand around your left index finger and hold it for a few minutes (Fig. 2-5), then wrap your hand around your right index finger and hold it for a few minutes (Fig. 2-6). Holding the index finger supports the following issues: timidity, mental confusion, depression, perfectionism, criticism, frustration, digestion, elimination, and wrist, elbow, and upperarm discomforts (Burmeister, 1994).

Figure 2-6   The quickie index finger – fear (right hand).

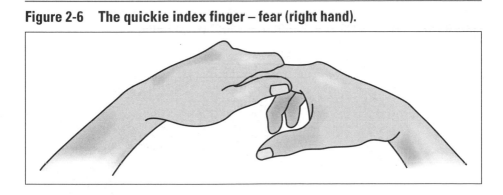

Figure 2-7   The quickie middle finger – anger (left hand).

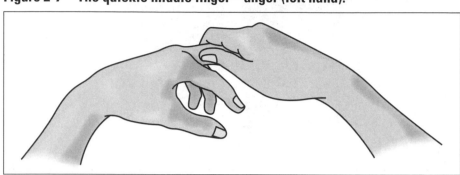

Benefits of self-care:

- Helps alleviate tooth discomfort.
- Improves problems with digestion.
- Helps with joint discomfort.
- Helps with back projects.
- Supports self-esteem and fear projects.

Description: Middle finger

The middle finger is used to represent anger in many cultures (and is often used in traffic jams). When people are unhappy with themselves or others, the imbalance manifests itself in this finger. For this exercise, simply wrap your hand around your left middle finger and hold it for a few minutes (Fig. 2-7), then wrap your hand around your right middle finger and hold it for a few minutes (Fig. 2-8). Holding the middle finger supports the following issues: feeling cowardly, irritable, indecisive, unstable, not alert, or overly emotional; general fatigue; eye problems; and forehead discomforts (Burmeister, 1994).

Figure 2-8   The quickie middle finger – anger (right hand).

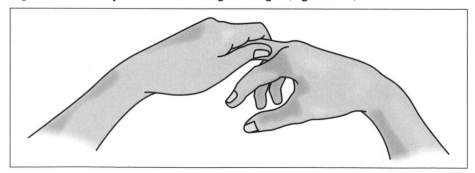

Figure 2-9   The quickie ring finger – sadness/grief (left hand).

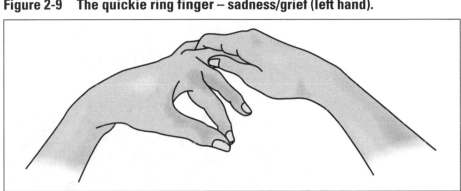

Benefits of self-care:

- Balances energy.
- Helps support vision issues.
- Balances lactation issues.
- Helps frontal headache issues.
- Balances out indecisiveness.
- Helps with anger management.

Description: Ring finger

The ring finger represents sadness and grief. Wedding rings are traditionally worn on this finger. This finger symbolizes our attachments to others and material possessions. When we lose these things or a relationship ends, we become sad and grieve over our losses. For this exercise, simply wrap your hand around your left ring finger and hold it for a few minutes (Fig. 2-9), then wrap your hand around your right ring finger and hold it for a few minutes (Fig. 2-10). Holding the ring

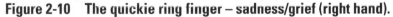

Figure 2-10   The quickie ring finger – sadness/grief (right hand).

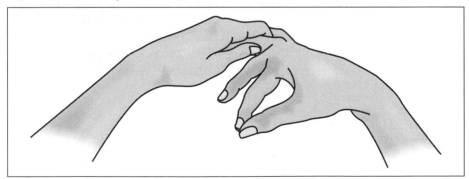

Figure 2-11   The quickie pinky finger – trying too hard (left hand).

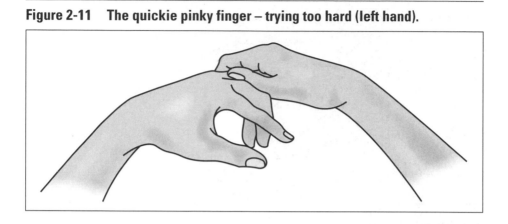

finger supports the following issues: negativity, mucus formation, and common sense (Burmeister, 1994).

Benefits of self-care:

- Supports respiratory issues.
- Supports tinnitus projects.
- Supports skin projects.
- Alleviates excessive congestion.
- Helps alleviate grief, negativity, and sadness.

Description: Pinky finger

The pinky finger represents pretense or trying too hard. Picture a tea party with little girls. They are sipping tea and pretending to be women. They are gossiping about things they know very little bit about, fantasizing, and playing the role of grown women they have observed. For this exercise, simply wrap your hand around your left pinky finger and hold it for a few minutes (Fig. 2-11), then wrap your hand around your right pinky finger and hold it for a few minutes (Fig. 2-12). Holding the pinky finger supports the following issues: "crying on the inside and laughing on the outside"; feeling insecure, nervous, or confused; "Why am I here?" issues; nervousness; and bloating (Burmeister, 1994).

Benefits of self-care:

- Supports heart conditions.
- Alleviates bloating, water imbalances.
- Alleviates anxiety.

Figure 2-12   The quickie pinky finger – trying too hard (right hand).

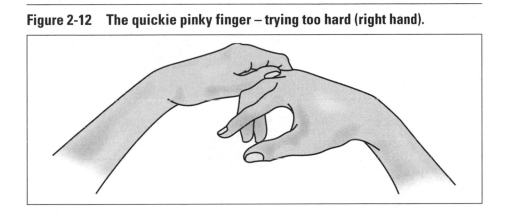

- Helps keep one from trying too hard.
- Helps keep one from being judgmental.

Steps for the Longer Sequence: (The Quickie steps are reiterated for review)

Left hand

1. Wrap the four fingers of your right hand around the left thumb. Breathe slowly as you do this.* (Wait until you feel a pulse before you go to the next finger. If your finger is already pulsating strongly, hold the finger until the pulsation has calmed down considerably). The sequence is thumb, middle finger, little finger (Fig. 2-13).

Figure 2-13   The thumb sequence (left hand).

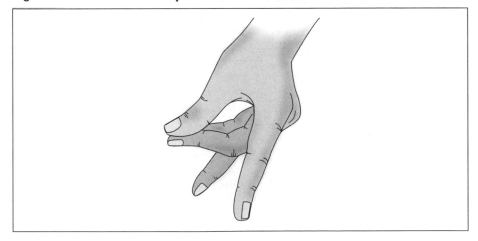

Figure 2-14   The index finger sequence (left hand).

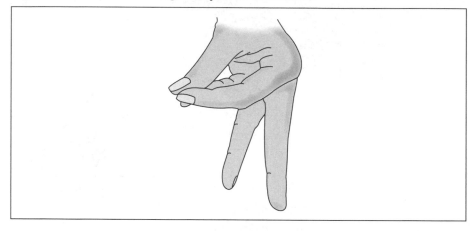

2. Wrap the four fingers of your right hand around your left index finger.* The sequence is thumb, index finger, little finger (Fig. 2-14).
3. Wrap the four fingers of your right hand around your left middle finger.* The sequence is little finger, ring finger, middle finger (Fig. 2-15).
4. Wrap the four fingers of your right hand around your left ring finger.* The sequence is thumb, index finger, middle finger, ring finger (Fig. 2-16).
5. Wrap the four fingers of your right hand around your left little finger.* The sequence is little finger, ring finger (Fig. 2-17).

Figure 2-15   The middle finger sequence (left hand).

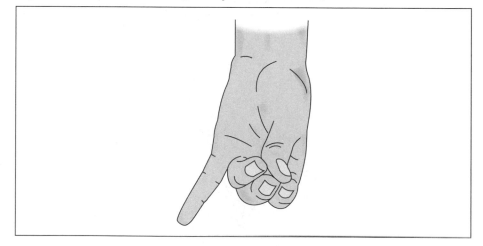

Figure 2-16   The ring finger sequence (left hand).

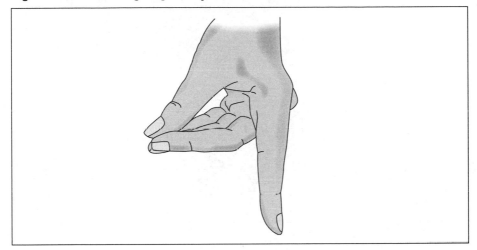

Figure 2-17   The pinky finger sequence (left hand).

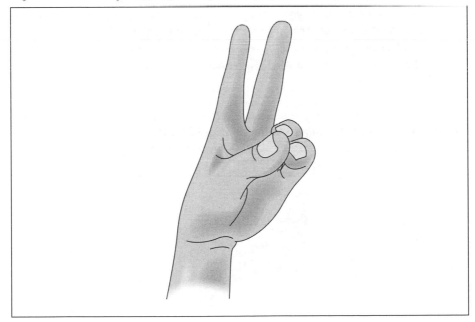

Figure 2-18   The thumb sequence (right hand).

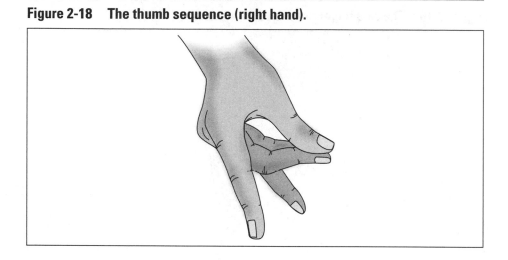

Right hand (the longer sequence used for the left hand is the same for the right hand also)

1. Wrap the four fingers of your left hand around your right thumb. Breathe slowly as you do this. The longer thumb sequence is shown in Figure 2-18.
2. Wrap the four fingers of your left hand around your right index finger. Breathe slowly as you do this. The longer index sequence is shown in Figure 2-19.
3. Wrap the four fingers of your left hand around your right middle finger. Breathe slowly as you do this. The longer middle finger sequence is shown in Figure 2-20.

Figure 2-19   The index finger sequence (right hand).

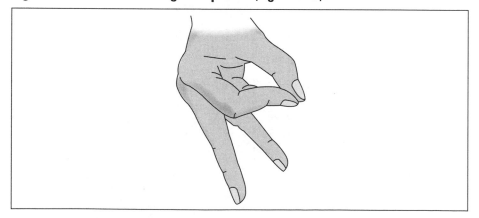

Figure 2-20   The middle finger sequence (right hand).

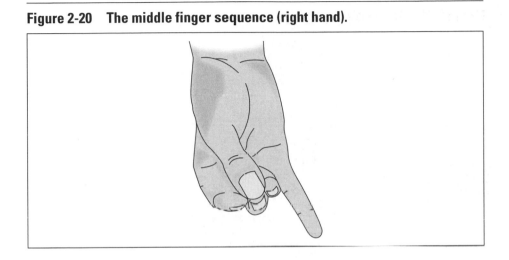

4. Wrap the four fingers of your left hand around your right ring finger. Breathe slowly as you do this. The longer ring finger sequence is shown in Figure 2-21.
5. Wrap the four fingers of your left hand around your right little finger. Breathe slowly as you do this. The longer little finger sequence is shown in Figure 2-22.
6. Take your left hand and hold your right palm.

Figure 2-21   The ring finger sequence (right hand).

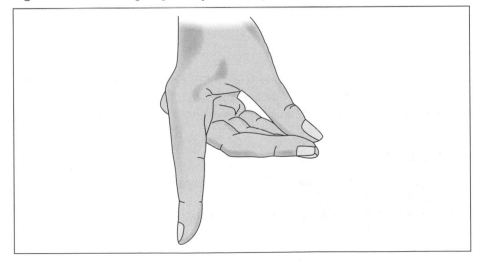

Figure 2-22   The pinky finger sequence (right hand).

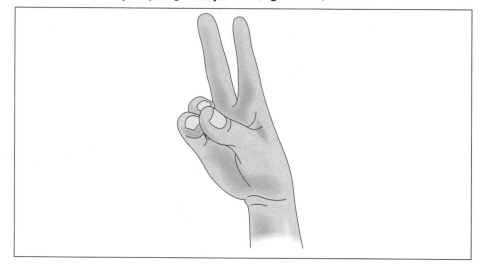

Mudras or Finger Poses

Description:

During his illness, Master Jiro Murai explored many finger positions that helped clear various blockages he had within his body. These finger positions work to achieve a purpose of balance and harmony within the body, and can provide relief for you in any situation. You can perform the exercises while you're sitting, lying down, chatting with patients, or watching television. Your hands are tools that you carry with you everywhere you go.

The Steps:

Finger Pose 1

Exhaling the burdens and blockages (Fig. 2-23). Hold the palm side of your left middle finger lightly with your right thumb. Place the rest of your right fingers on the back of your left middle finger. (This can be reversed for the right middle finger.)

Benefits of self-care:

- Supports us in our exhalation process so we can empty ourselves of blocked energy.
- General tension is released from the head to toe.
- Supports vision.

Figure 2-23   Exhaling burdens and blockages.

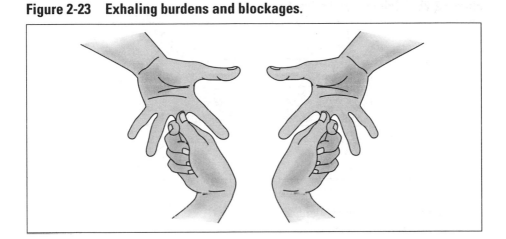

- Helps with indecisiveness and procrastination.
- Alleviates fatigue in the body.

Finger Pose 2

Inhaling abundance (Fig. 2-24). Hold the back of your left middle finger lightly with your right thumb. Place the rest of your right fingers on the palm side of your left middle finger. (This can be reversed for the right middle finger.)

Benefits of self-care:

- Supports inhaling deeply.
- Supports vision projects.

Figure 2-24   Inhaling abundance.

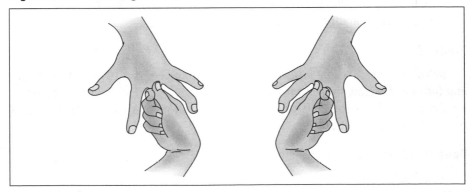

Figure 2-25   Calming and revitalizing.

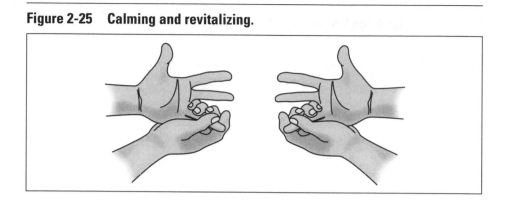

- Helps with hearing challenges.
- Supports foot projects.
- Supports clarity and alertness.

Finger Pose 3

Calming and revitalizing (Fig. 2-25). Hold the palm side of your left little and ring fingers with your right thumb. Place the rest of your right fingers on the back of your left little and ring fingers. (This can be reversed for the right hand.)

Benefits of self-care:

- Calms the body.
- Releases nervous tension and stress.
- Revitalizes all organ functions.
- Alleviates nervousness.
- Alleviates worry about the heart.
- Helps with short-windedness.
- Helps keep one from trying too hard.
- Helps with inability to enjoy life.

Finger Pose 4

Releasing general daily fatigue (Fig. 2-26). Hold the back of your left thumb and index and middle fingers with your right thumb. Place the rest of your fingers on the palm side of your left thumb and index and middle fingers. (This can be reversed for the right thumb and fingers.)

Benefits of self-care:

- Releases fatigue.
- Releases tension and stress that build up during the course of the day.

Figure 2-26 Releasing general daily fatigue.

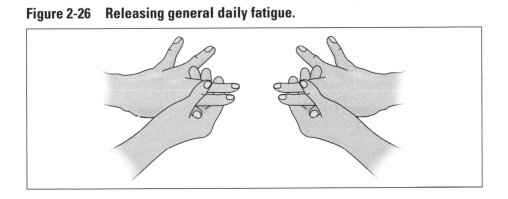

- Helps release worry, fear, and anger.
- Alleviates insecurity regarding career, money, relationships.
- Helps with feeling and looking old.
- Helps keep one from being overly sensitive and easily agitated.
- Helps keep one from being a worrywart.

Finger Pose 5

Total revitalization (Fig. 2-27). Make a circle with your right middle finger and thumb (palm side of thumb on middle fingernail). Next, slip your left thumb between the circle of your right thumb and middle finger (left thumb palm touching right middle fingernail). (This can be reversed for the right thumb.)

Benefits of self-care:

- Rejuvenates the body's functions.
- Clears the blockages causing daily fatigue.

Figure 2-27 Total revitalization.

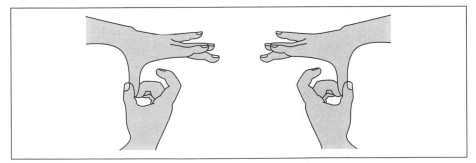

- Settles feelings of unrest.
- Balances feelings of tiredness for no reason.
- Helps calm edginess.
- Curbs sweet-tooth cravings.

Finger Pose 6

Breathing easily (Fig. 2-28). Touch your ring fingernail with the palm side of your thumb (can be done on both hands).

Benefits of self-care:

- Strengthens the respiratory system and function.
- Helps support ear projects.
- Facilitates easier breathing during exercise.
- Supports altitude changes when traveling to high altitudes.
- Helps with skin conditions.
- Helps with feelings of rejection.
- Reduces ditzy, careless, or clumsy behaviors.
- Helps to restore good sense.

Figure 2-28   Breathing easily.

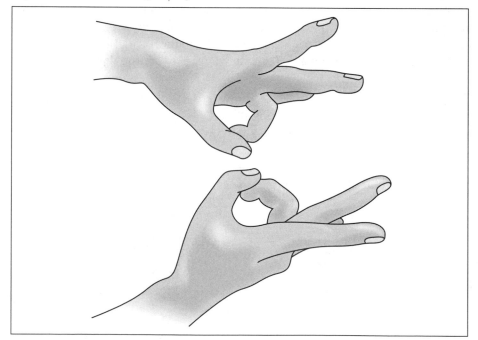

Figure 2-29 Exhaling dirt, dust, and greasy grime.

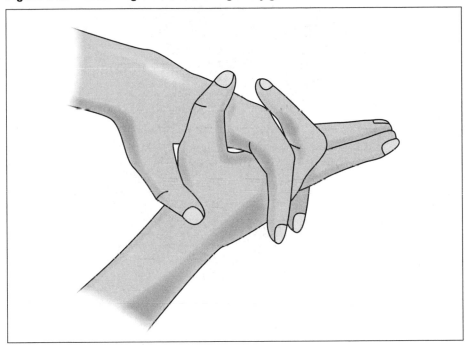

Finger Pose 7

Exhaling dirt, dust, and greasy grime (Fig. 2-29). Touch the palms of your left and right middle fingers in a folded-hands position (make a church steeple with your middle fingers).

Benefits of self-care:

- Reinforces the exhalation process.
- Releases general daily tension and stress from the head.
- Supports the lungs.
- Supports digestive functions.
- Supports the abdomen.
- Supports the legs.

Finger Pose 8

Inhaling the purified breath of life (Fig. 2-30). Touch your left middle finger-nail with your right middle fingernail.

Figure 2-30   Inhaling the purified breath of life.

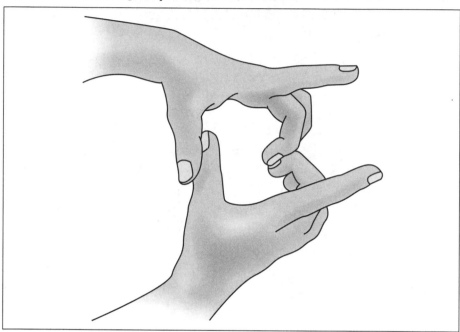

Benefits of self-care:

- Releases tension in the back.
- Promotes overall feeling of well-being.
- Strengthens the ability to breathe in the purified breath of life.

EXPERIENCING JIN SHIN JYUTSU® AS A CLIENT

Selecting a Practitioner

If you have never experienced a Jin Shin Jyutsu session before, I suggest a visit to the Jin Shin Jyutsu Web site. The practitioner directory allows you to search your geographical location for a practitioner, and includes only those who have met the criteria for being a practitioner and/or self-help instructor. If you find a practitioner outside of this directory, you should ask to see his or her certificate. If a certificate cannot be produced, for any reason, you might want to consider verifying the legitimacy of your potential practitioner with the Jin Shin Jyutsu office.

Pricing for Sessions

The average price for a 1-hour session ranges from $65 to $85.

Duration and Frequency of Sessions

A typical Jin Shin Jyutsu session is about 45 minutes to 1.5 hours long. The frequency of the sessions depends on the health challenge involved. With chronic illnesses and acute conditions, the sessions will vary in time and duration. Children, animals, and people with more severe illnesses often require less time. Animals and children tend to be more simple and open to healing, where an average adult might have a harder time relaxing so that blockages can be released. People who are more ill often require less time, but more frequent sessions depending on the case. In people who are more ill, it can be a great deal of work when the body is working to regain harmony and the body can feel tired more quickly, especially when there are many blockages to work through. More sessions and shorter times can help a person who is more ill from feeling more worn out during the healing process. More serious issues usually require more sessions. The practitioner begins to taper down when necessary, but also teaches self-care immediately and in an ongoing fashion.

What to Expect From a Session

The practitioner does his or her own private preparation for your arrival. This may include saying a prayer, setting intentions for the visit, or simply meditating. The session is conducted with your clothes on; however, it is recommended that you remove your shoes and any restrictive clothing. Dress comfortably initially (sweats or loose clothes are always comfortable). Take an extra blanket (although usually the practitioner will have one), just in case you get a little chilly. You will have a heightened sensitivity to temperature changes when you experience energy work. As the client, you will be lying on your back on a massage table of some sort. However, no massage or manipulations like those you might receive from a chiropractor or osteopath are involved, and no drugs, chemicals, or substances are used during the session. Aromatherapy or music may be used, depending on the preferences of you and your practitioner. The practitioner will gently touch various parts of your body with his or her fingertips, while you remain totally clothed. You will experience the practitioner's hands shifting around to different parts of your body at different times. Don't try to make sense of it. Just relax. The results experienced from the session should be those of stress reduction and relaxation from the daily tensions of the day, promoting overall harmony and balance in your life.

Self-Help Classes

Another great way to nurture yourself is to participate in self-help classes. The classes are usually informal and are led by Jin Shin Jyutsu practitioners in the area. They trade sessions with one another and discuss various things relating to what they are studying or learning in Jin Shin Jyutsu. These community groups gather at designated places such as homes, churches, or community centers. They are generally open to new faces. Check with the Jin Shin Jyutsu headquarters to find a self-help group in your area. There may also be a self-help class you can you can take once you meet the requirements. Taking such a class enables you to teach self-help classes in the community.

Further Studies in Jin Shin Jyutsu

Classes and Certification

- After completing the 5-day basic seminar, you will be given a certificate for 35 hours of class time and participation. This is a certificate of completion.
- After attending the 5-day basic seminar three times, you will be awarded a certificate for 105 hours of class time and participation. Completing these three classes gives you the opportunity to become a Jin Shin Jyutsu Student Practitioner and begin a lifelong study of Jin Shin Jyutsu. We are always students; therefore, the Student Practitioner title remains throughout the study course.

Special Classes

- In special classes, students learn how to teach others to care for themselves using Jin Shin Jyutsu. The Living the Art Seminar is open to individuals who have completed the 5-day basic seminar three times. The course explores the practice of self-help and daily maintenance that moves us toward self-sufficiency and personal empowerment in our health care. Students engage in sharing self-help with others in their family, at work, and in community settings. This class enables a practitioner to teach self-help to others, in accordance with the self-help books specially written by Mary Burmeister.
- An advanced-level course is the Now Know Myself Seminar, which explores Jin Shin Jyutsu Texts 1 and 2 in further detail. Students are required to have attended the 5-day seminar three times. With this course, students can deepen their understanding of the art, and gain new perspectives on the concepts previously taught.

- A Student/Practitioner Mentoring program is offered at the main office in Arizona. This program enables students to gather in a small group setting with an experienced instructor. They can participate in discussions, hands-on activities, and study activities that will facilitate their growth as practitioners. The program lasts a week (7 hours a day), and participants are required to have taken the 5-day basic seminar five times (or either the 5-day basic seminar four times or the Now Know Myself, Living the Art, or two Special Topic classes over a 3-year period).
- The following is a list of many of the Special Topic classes that are taught throughout the United States and other countries:
  - Pulses
  - Body Reading
  - The Depths
  - The Methods of Correction
  - Astrology
  - Organ Flows

These classes require the attendance of one 5-day basic seminar, unless otherwise specified.

The tuition for each class varies and does not include lodging or travel. Exact pricing can be found on the Jin Shin Jyutsu Web site (contact information is provided). There is a reduced price for classes that the student is repeating. If there are no practitioners in your area, you might consider taking a road trip and attending the class elsewhere, and/or gathering a group of interested people in your area who might want to form a class. The Jin Shin Jyutsu office will be happy to work with you to coordinate a seminar in your area.

Contact Information

Jin Shin Jyutsu, Inc.
8719 E. San Alberto Drive
Scottsdale, AZ 85258
Phone: 480-998-9331
Fax: 480-998-9335
http://www.jsjinc.net

REFERENCES

Burmeister, M. (1994). *Introducing Jin Shin Jyutsu Is: Book I*. Scottsdale, AZ: Jin Shin Jyutsu, Inc.

Burmeister, A., & Monte, T. (1997). *The touch of healing*. New York: Bantam Books.

Merriam-Webster online dictionary. Retrieved March 16, 2009, from http://www.merriam-webster.com/dictionary/art

SUGGESTED READING LIST

Burmeister, M. (1981). *Introducing Jin Shin Jyutsu Is: Book II*. Scottsdale, AZ: Jin Shin Jyutsu, Inc.

Burmeister, M. (1985). *Introducing Jin Shin Jyutsu Is: Book III*. Scottsdale, AZ: Jin Shin Jyutsu, Inc.

Pflueger, L. (1997). *What Mary says, . . .* Scottsdale, AZ: Jin Shin Jyutsu, Inc.

Sempell, P. (2000 April/May). Jin Shin Jyutsu and modern medicine: Integrating the ancient healing art of Jin Shin Jyutsu with modern medicine of heart transplants. *Massage and Bodywork*, 1–8.

Peters, M. (2007 July). Japanese acupressure technique targets blocked energy. Available at: http://seattlepi.nwsource.com/health/322345_hcenter05.html. Accessed October 28, 2009.

CHAPTER 3

Reiki: Life Force Energy for Self-Care

RACHEL Y. HILL

The Five Reiki Principles

Just for today I will accept my many blessings. Just for today I will trust.
Just for today I will be at peace. Just for today I will do my work honestly.
Just for today I will respect the rights of all life forms.

—DR. MIKAO USUI

INTRODUCTION TO USUI REIKI

The term Reiki is pronounced "ray-key," and thus sounds like rake, the garden tool we use to clean up leaves. When I first learned of this healing modality, I imagined myself using a garden rake to smooth someone's energy field out. The image I had in my mind was a little scary. I was a little puzzled about how this raking device would work. I was hoping the instructors would have a smaller rake I could use, because a bigger garden rake would probably scare my clients away! I was very much relieved when I learned Reiki was nothing like a garden tool. I could leave my garden tools exactly where they were. Reiki is a form of energy therapy in which healing and balance are achieved by the placement of hands over selected positions on an individual's body.

Although Reiki is similar to many energy therapies, it is differentiated by the way in which a person is able to share the technique with others. Reiki students are attuned or initiated (the chakras are opened and balanced to channel this special energy) by their Reiki Master Teacher to practice Reiki on themselves and on others. Special symbols that were imparted to Dr. Mikao Usui are used to activate the healing sequences during treatments, and to open and balance the chakras of the student so that he or she can share Reiki with others. Once you are attuned to Reiki, you become part of a lineage that can be traced back to the original Reiki Master Teachers. When we practice energy medicine with individuals, we learn many techniques that help to shift and move energy around to restore balance. We can become very skilled and attuned to use our intuition and manipulate the energy field with our understanding of the healing process. With Reiki, we are allowing the chi, ki, prana, pneuma, or life force energy to go where it is needed in a person's body. Basically, we relieve ourselves of the responsibility to make anything happen. We simply place our hands on the body positions and allow the life force energy to go where it needs to go to help the individual who is receiving treatment. Many practitioners in other modalities also practice Reiki, and believe that the Reiki attunements they receive heighten the other forms of healing that they practice with others. Since I have been studying Reiki, I can feel a difference in the touch I share with others. Before I learned Reiki, I would do different healing work with patients and individuals, and it would take a little time before things would get cooking or I could actually feel the energy start to move in my hands. Since I've become attuned to Reiki, my hands begin to heat up before I even touch the person I am working on. I have been doing energy work for the past 11 years now, so I suspect that the action of constantly connecting with others also intensifies the heat being generated in my hands. I don't want to give the impression that I am on autopilot, but in a way I am. The life force is the pilot and I am just a channel for the energy. I remove my desires for any specific outcomes from the situation and step aside for the highest good to be done for my client and for myself. I just let the life force energy do what it needs to do.

Reiki is not associated with any religion. I have been approached in the healthcare setting by healthcare providers with strong religious convictions. They often have legitimate questions about such terms as "life force energy," "universal energy," and "channeling of the life force energy." I always like to reassure them that I don't impose my religious beliefs on anyone, and that the universal life force (which may seem foreign to them) is simply the breath of life that has kept humanity going since creation. I believe strongly that the healing that took place in biblical times was very much related to the knowledge we once lost and are now regaining through the reemergence of these energetic healing modalities.

History of Usui Reiki

Dr. Mikao Usui

Much of the story of how Reiki was rediscovered has been passed down through oral tradition. There are also several versions of this story. I have chosen what resonates with me as a student, teacher, and practitioner of Reiki. The Usui system of Reiki is named after its founder, Dr. Mikao Usui. According to oral history, Dr. Usui was an educator in Kyoto, Japan in the late 1800s. He began an investigation of the healing phenomena of history's greatest spiritual teachers. Through travel, study, research, and meditation, he developed the healing practice of Reiki and spent the rest of his life applying and teaching this method.

The Usui system of Reiki healing was spread by individuals who participated in the tradition of teaching, sharing information, and exchanging treatments. The original story I was told was that Dr. Usui's students asked him about the works of Christ and why no one had been able to do greater works, as Jesus had mentioned. Dr. Usui was unable to answer that question, so he left the school and set out to find the answers that were unavailable to his students and to himself. His quest lasted about 10 years, during which time he sought answers through Buddhism. The Buddhist monks told him that the teachings he sought had been lost; therefore, the only way to find answers would be to seek enlightenment. It has been said that Dr. Usui spent 7 years in the United States, hoping to find the answers from Christians, and that he entered the Chicago School of Divinity; however, there is no record of that journey (Stein, 1995). It is possible that these stories were created to make Reiki more acceptable in the West, because the concepts were unlike what we have been accustomed to accepting or comprehending. After studying the Christian literature, Dr. Usui returned to complete his studies at a Zen monastery. There he found texts with different formulas for healing. He taught himself to read in Sanskrit, but was unable to activate the symbols and formulas he discovered. In an attempt to decipher the formulas and unlock the answers, Dr. Usui went on a 21-day quest. He went to Mt. Koriyama in Japan. He took 21 stones with him to track the time, and fasted and meditated for 21 days. After each day, he would throw a stone to mark the time. On the final morning of his quest, Dr. Usui was hit in the forehead by a beam of light. He lost consciousness for a bit, but regained his senses and experienced a vision of millions of bubbles. The symbols used for Reiki today appeared to him. As they appeared, he received the formulas for each of them to activate the healing energy they held. He had been attuned to the Reiki energy. He left Mt. Koriyama and encountered what we know in Reiki history as the four miracles. The first miracle occurred when Dr. Usui was walking down the mountain and hurt his toe. When he held his toe in his hand, it was instantly healed. The second miracle happened when he went to a little house and was given a full meal and did not get sick after fasting for 21 days. The woman who served him the meal had a terrible toothache, which Dr. Mikao healed. This was the third miracle. The final miracle was the healing of the director of the monastery, who was suffering an attack of arthritis. Dr. Usui called this healing method Reiki (Stein, 1995. Reiki is the life force energy that comes through us to help others to heal. Dr. Usui knew that the healing power that came through him was not of his own doing but of a much greater power. He set out to heal the poorest people in the area and spent his life serving others and teaching Reiki. He found that when he treated people, they were not always appreciative or ready to be completely healed. For example, if a person is blind and is able to collect enough money in a cup to eat for a day or a week, what happens when his or her eyes are healed? He or she is placed in a situation of change and must get a job to provide for himself or herself, and transition from their old way of being. Some are happy about the change, but some are ungrateful and feel they were better off in their old state. I have seen this behavior in myself before, and even in patients I have cared for. I have found myself stuck in a comfort zone, and when I am free, I have to find another excuse for myself. You can only be healed when you are truly ready. Dr. Usui learned that people appreciate Reiki more if they give some form of payment, no matter how small, in exchange for the healings they receive. He died in 1930, having trained about 18 Reiki Masters. Dr. Chujiro Hayashi is probably the most popular Master trained by Dr. Usui, because he is the only one who has been documented in any of the Reiki sources we have today.

Mrs. Hawayo Takata

Mrs. Hawayo Takata was born in 1900 to a family of sugarcane workers or (according to some stories) pineapple cutters on the island of Kauai, Hawaii, at Hanamaulu. She wasn't strong enough to work on the plantations, so she worked as a fountain clerk and in the school system helping young children. She married a plantation accountant and was very happy. They had two daughters together. However, he died of a heart attack at the age of 32. She was very ill and financially devastated, and found herself raising two small children alone. Then her sister passed away as well, and she needed to go back to Tokyo and carry word to her parents (who had moved back to Japan). She was able to gather up enough money to take a cattle boat to Japan; however, the journey weakened her more. She apparently had gall bladder issues that required surgery, but she was far too weak for that. She also had respiratory problems that doctors feared would be fatal if they used anesthesia on her. As the story goes, she developed appendicitis in addition to all her other physical ailments. The night before the surgery, she heard a voice saying, "The surgery is not necessary." While she was being prepped for surgery, she heard the voice again. She asked her doctor if there was another way she could experience healing. The doctor told her there was another way and referred her to Chujiro Hayashi's Reiki clinic.

Mrs. Takata was able to experience healing from the benefits of Reiki and enjoyed her healing for months. She worked tirelessly to persuade Dr. Hayashi to teach her the technique. Some say he refused at first because she was a woman, and others say it was because he was not ready for Reiki to leave Japan at that time. Nevertheless, in 1936 she was taught Reiki I, and in 1937 she was taught Reiki II. She worked in the clinic and lived in Japan for 2 years after that. She became a massage therapist and opened her first clinic in Kapaa. In 1938, Dr. Hayashi visited Mrs. Takata in Hawaii and attuned her to Reiki III. He was very impressed with her commitment to healing others, and her persistence won him over. It is said that he announced her as his successor and gave her clear instructions to not give Reiki training away without a charge (Stein, 1995).

Mrs. Takata went on to teach Reiki in the United States. During the first 30 years, she only taught Reiki I and Reiki II to others. It wasn't until the last decade of her life that she created 22 Reiki Masters. She felt that only those who were dedicated to a lifetime of studying and practicing Reiki would be fit to be Masters. She did not have financial problems anymore because she was able to make an abundant living teaching Reiki. She charged $10,000 for training, which was her effort to weed out the students who were less committed. She lectured only—notes and recordings were not allowed in her class. The oral tradition was definitely the means by which Reiki had been taught originally, and that tradition was continued by Mrs. Takata.

Dr. Chujiro Hayashi

In 1925, at the age of 47, Dr. Chujiro Hayashi received his Master's training. At the time of his death, he had become the successor to the Reiki ministry. He had opened a clinic in Tokyo, trained 16 Masters, and worked on numerous people in need of healing. He and his students also made house calls to visit those who were sick and unable to make it to the clinic. It is said that on May 10, 1941, Chujiro Hayashi stopped his heart by psychic means and made his transition. He predicted World War II and knew that Reiki would no longer be available in Japan. Eventually the center was taken over, just as he had foretold. It was through Mrs. Takata that the Reiki concept was able to live on.

Concept of Usui Reiki

The word Reiki consists of two Japanese words: *rei*, meaning the higher power, universal life force, or spirit; and *ki*, meaning the energy found in every living being. Joined together, the words mean "universal life energy." Reiki is based on the premise that illness is a result of some energetic disruption in the body. Reiki consists of four levels that range from beginner to teacher. At each level the individual is a practioner. Each level creates a foundation for the practioner that bridges to the next level. The Reiki practitioner helps to improve the flow of energy and release blockages that exist in the energetic system of the body, to help alleviate pain, discomfort, and illnesses that have arisen. The practitioner uses his or her hands to pass the Reiki energy on to the client. Because the Reiki energy is coming from a higher source, the connection with the client raises his or her vibration to that of the healing life force energy. Tuning forks have a neat way of resonating with other tuning forks. When you strike a "C" tuning fork, hold it up to another tuning fork. Listen to what begins to happen. You have tuning forks resonating with one another. This is how healing and relief take place in many healing modalities, not just Reiki. There are usually about 13 to 16 different hand positions in Reiki, depending on how it has been taught. As with many other modalities, it is not a coincidence that the major chakras of the body are covered in the hand positions used in Reiki. The practitioner goes through the various hand positions, allows the energy to flow, and moves to the next position when he or she intuitively feels it is time to go on.

Terms Related to Usui Reiki

Attunement – An initiation by which the Reiki Master Teacher enters the energy field/aura of his or her students and prepares the chakras in their body to receive the universal Reiki energy that will allow them to help bring balance to others.

Aura – An emanation of subtle energy from the body that can be utilized to detect various states of physical, mental, and emotional health.

Chakras – Sacred wheels or energy centers of the body that are extensions of the aura; each relates to specific organs and glands of the body, and can be utilized to detect imbalances in the body, mind, and spirit.

Energy healing – Using energy from an outside source to create a change that promotes harmony and balance within one's body or that of another individual.

Hand positions – There are 16 hand positions in the Usui Reiki System that are used to achieve balance within the body.

Lineage – The listed (or unlisted) legacy of attunements that have preceded a student who has become attuned to Reiki (with his or her teacher preceding him or her).

Oku Den – Reiki level 2, or second-degree Reiki. This level explores the mental and emotional aspects of self-care, and expands on the physical self-care of oneself and others. The attunement of this level allows one to treat others.

Reiki – Rei is the Christ or Buddha consciousness, and Ki is the universal life force energy.

Reiki principles – Five principles to live by that can help one lead a healthier, more balanced life.

1. Just for today I will accept my many blessings.
2. Just for today I will trust.
3. Just for today I will be at peace.
4. Just for today I will do my work honestly.
5. Just for today I will respect the rights of all life forms.

Reiki symbols – Secret symbols used in Reiki for healing that can help energize the session, facilitate mental and emotional healing, and allow the practitioner to help others from a distance.

Sensei – Japanese title that is used to address teachers, professors, and other professionals such as doctors and attorneys.

Shinpiden – Reiki level 3 or Master levels, meaning mystery teaching. This level accommodates the exploration and healing of oneself and others on spiritual, physical, mental, and emotional levels. The Master level and Master Teacher level are both included in this category.

Shoden – Reiki level 1 or first degree, used primarily for the care of one's own physical body or that of others, promoting self-healing and exploring one's own potential to heal.

Subtle energy – Faint electromagnetic energy fields that exist within living creatures.

Universal life force energy – The energy that is active within every living being.

REIKI SELF-CARE PRACTICES

If you are just now learning about Reiki and are not currently a practitioner, you should not practice self-care on yourself. You could try, but the energy you generate would not be as effective and would come from something other than the life force energy. This could increase your risk of being drained and tired if you try to conduct Reiki outside its natural process. You must be attuned to the Reiki energy in order to provide care to yourself and to others. Don't worry. You can experience Reiki whether you are attuned or not. You can experience self-care either through a practitioner or in Reiki Circles, where practitioners gather to share Reiki with others. Another way to obtain self-care is to take a Reiki I or II class, which will attune you to the Reiki energy that allows you to practice on yourself and others. If you choose this route and know other nurses who are practitioners, you can create a network and share Reiki with one another. Remember that not being attuned does not keep you from experiencing the benefits of Reiki. Use the alternative self-care options given, and enjoy the experience.

Experiencing the Five Principles of Reiki

The Five Principles of Reiki were most likely created by Dr. Mikao Usui and are considered the Reiki commandments that practitioners strive to live by. Each principle is very powerful and is a way in which any compassionate human would want to lead his or her life anyway. The principles may present a challenge for us in some way, to abandon old ways of thinking that prevent us from being the best we can be at home, at work, or in our relationships with others. By practicing each principle, we explore the opportunities for us to overcome these challenges and realize our potential so that we can care for ourselves in the deepest way possible. The principles hold a key to establishing balance in all aspects of our lives. Each one takes practice and dedication. Read and study the five principles of Reiki. Explore what each principle means to you and how it can be applied to real-life situations you are facing. How can these principles be applied each day, at work, at home, and in everyday interactions with others? Keep a journal to record your experience and any insights you may have. Share these insights with others, if you are participating in a group. If you are working alone, reflect on the principles as often and frequently as you are led to.

Reiki Principle 1: Just for today I will accept my many blessings

It is not surprising how much we are able to receive when we feel gratitude for what we already have at work or at home. Working in a healthcare setting, we can easily become accustomed to seeing sick and dying people every day. We forget how quickly life and health can slip from our grasp. The act of gratitude itself makes us much more attentive to what we have right now, in this moment. Gratitude is powerful enough to stimulate the flow of abundance and ongoing blessings in our lives daily, keeping us thankful and harmonious with our surroundings.

Reiki Principle 2: Just for today I will trust

When we are unable to trust in the divine order of things, our only other option is to worry. This poses a challenge for us in the healthcare setting because we don't always understand why things happen as they do. Why do children have to die, why does a patient with leukemia in remission experience its sudden return, why do we have challenging work situations that have no immediate solution? Things can often look grim and terrible; however, you can shift your thoughts and emotions, and choose to feel something different. In doing so, you conserve energy that you were sending to fear and doubt. You invite a great deal of light to shine on the experience and change it for the better.

Reiki Principle 3: Just for today I will be at peace

How many opportunities arise in a day for us to be angry about something, someone, or some event that did or didn't work out? However, anger never resolves any situation we experience, nor does carrying anger around allow us to be who we truly are. John Lennon once sang a song with a famous chorus: "All we are saying is give peace a chance." It's ironic that he was killed by a gunshot from another person. However, his message and his words ring on. When you have a choice to be mad, find something in the situation to be glad about.

Reiki Principle 4: Just for today I will do my work honestly

There are many opportunities to be unethical in the healthcare setting. We see it in billing for services, insurance claims, substance abuse, fudging on time sheets, padding mileage, and in sharing our true feelings with others. It is a reality that people will consider acting dishonestly. There are many times when we feel like we have done a good job at the end of our day, but we should look at ourselves through the truest lens to know whether or not we truly are doing our best. In everything we do, integrity and morality should follow. This inner commitment comes from within and is a choice, as are all the other principles of Reiki.

Reiki Principle 5: Just for today I will respect the rights of all life forms

The healthcare setting is very diverse and grows more diverse by the day. There are so many races, cultures, and ethnic backgrounds involved that special classes in diversity are necessary so that we can fully meet the needs of the patients. Nurses are faced with a variety of situations that warrant a reevaluation. The underlying solution is based on the golden rule: "Do unto others as you would have them do unto you."

Reiki Circles

A Reiki Circle is a great way to learn about Reiki. This is usually a like-minded group of individuals who gather weekly, biweekly, or monthly, and perform Reiki on themselves and on others in the community in need of balance. Reiki Circles can be located on the Internet (look for listings of holistic health practitioners), by postings in New Age bookstores, and through Reiki organizations.

Experiencing Usui Reiki as a Client

Selecting a Practitioner

The best way to find a Reiki practitioner in your area is to contact a Reiki organization, search through local health practitioner listings on the Internet, or search postings in New Age bookstores. People will often refer practitioners to others based on personal experience, and by word of mouth and reputation in the community. Not every Reiki practitioner has an official degree or certification. He or she may not be a member of a Reiki Organization or a healthcare professional. This does not mean that he or she is not an excellent practitioner. Don't be afraid to ask for credentials, to see certificates, and talk to the practitioner to see if he or she is the right fit for you.

Pricing for Sessions

The price range for Reiki sessions ranges from $65 to $85 for an hour-long session. Reiki Circles generally only ask for donations to help pay the rent for the space used, to defray the cost refreshments and materials, or to make a contribution to another organization or charity. Inquire about this at the time you are seeking out places to experience Reiki.

Duration and Frequency of Sessions

Sessions generally last from 45 minutes to 1.5 hours. The frequency of treatment depends on what is occurring with the body. Acute conditions may warrant more frequent sessions, until things begin to stabilize and completely resolve. Elderly people, infants and children, and seriously ill clients don't usually require a full hour-long session. A shorter session will provide them with just as much benefit, without overloading their systems.

What to Expect From a Session

The practitioner might begin the session by checking your aura, by running his hand above the length of your body or by using a pendulum. The pendulum is a piece of wood, metal, or stone suspended from a string that can detect the pattern of your chakras. It can show the practitioner whether the chakras are moving in a normal or abnormal fashion. This information allows him to detect imbalances and disharmony in the body. There are 16 hand positions in which a Reiki practitioner places his hands on or directly above a specific area of the client's fully clothed body. The Reiki energy will flow, as previously mentioned, through the practitioner's hand into the client's body. There are many sensations that can be felt during a session, but if you feel nothing, it is still all right. The energetic transfer of the universal life force energy is often felt as a mild to moderate radiation of heat, coolness of the body, buzzing in different parts of the body, tingling, or weightedness. The client can actually have a variety of experiences, from recalling memories of the past to visiting unknown places. At the end of the session, your aura is swept clean with a brushing motion of the hands, down the length of your body. The general overall feeling is one of relaxation and peace. Reiki is a very cleansing practice; therefore, the ailment you're experiencing may seem to get worse before it begins to improve. Don't be discouraged; often the energy is just moving and the body is clearing itself. It is advisable to drink lots of fluid to help facilitate the cleansing process. Reiki does not replace consultations with a physician or health practitioner.

Reiki I and II Classes

Description of Reiki Self-Care Practice

To practice this self-care exercise, you must be attuned to the Reiki symbols. Taking a Reiki I or II class is a proactive form of self-care. You are investing in yourself by learning Reiki. This self-care tool is priceless because you can benefit yourself and others. Because this book is about self-care, it would be ideal for you to experience Reiki for yourself first. You may feel you are ready to take on the world, and be tempted to line up 10 or 15 appointments with friends to practice your new skills. You will want to share with others and feel the impact of the attunements. However, you should take this time to be gentle with yourself. Once you are attuned to Reiki, you will experience a multilevel cleansing of your body, mind, and spirit. This requires lots of water, rest, and self-reflection. Nurture yourself with self-care Reiki, allowing yourself to find a deeper meaning in your healing experience. I am pretty certain you will have purchased a journal by now. If not, a binder with notebook paper will suffice. Do note your experiences, questions, understandings, thoughts, fears, and anything that comes across your mind, because it is very important. The details of a taking a Reiki I or II class will be discussed further below.

Hand Positions for Reiki Self-Care Treatment

Steps:

Before beginning, brush or sweep down your body to begin clearing your energy field of debris and energetic dust bunnies that can be easily removed to facilitate the healing process.

Figures 3-1 through 3-5a illustrate the hand placements for the Reiki head positions.

Position #1 (Fig. 3-1): Place your hands over your face, covering your eyes.

Position #2 (Fig. 3-2): Place your hands over your cheeks and ears.

Figure 3-1   Reiki self-care position 1.

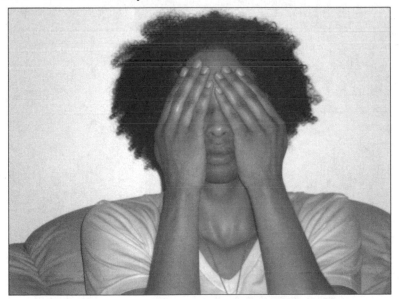

Figure 3-2   Reiki self-care position 2.

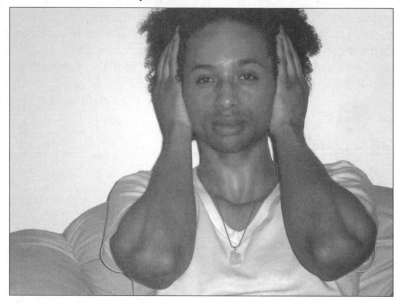

Figure 3-3   Reiki self-care position 3.

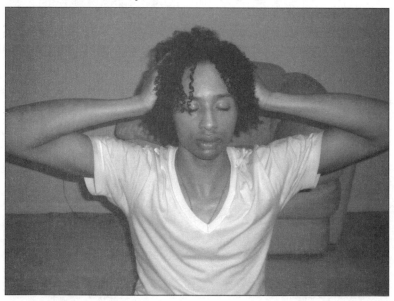

Figure 3-4   Reiki self-care position 4.

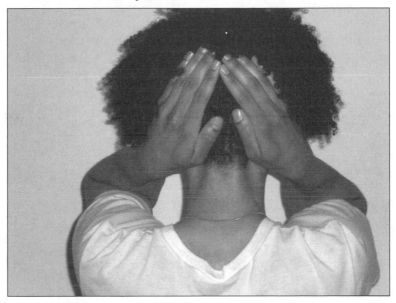

Figure 3-5a   Reiki self-care position 5a.

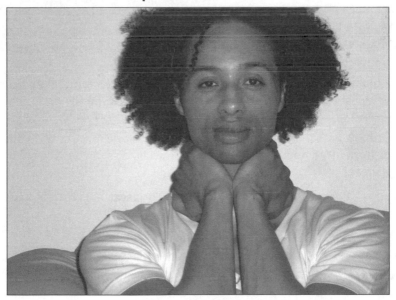

Figure 3-5b   Reiki self-care position 5b.

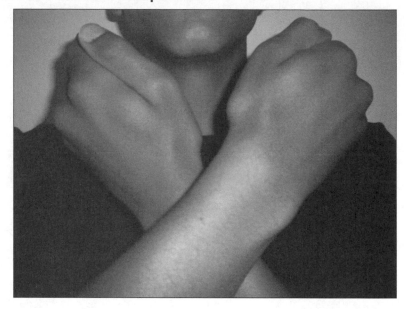

Position #3 (Fig. 3-3): Place your hands on top of your head with the fingers touching (but not overlapping).

Position #4 (Fig. 3-4): Place your hands on the back of your head over the occipital ridge.

Position #5a (Fig. 3-5a): Place the inside of both wrists together and cup your throat with your hands (with the fingers resting on the both sides of the neck).

Position #5b (Fig. 3-5b): An alternate position is to cup your hands and hold them in front of the throat (for those who can't tolerate touching in this area).

Figures 3-6 through 3-10 illustrate the hand placements for the Reiki trunk positions.

Position #6 (Fig. 3-6): Place both hands over your breastbone and heart area.

Position #7 (Fig. 3-7): Place both hands below your breast on the lower part of the ribcage.

Figure 3-6   Reiki self-care position 6.

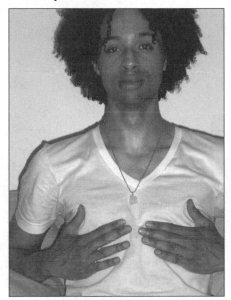

Figure 3-7   Reiki self-care position 7.

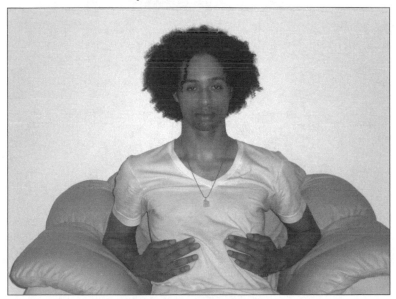

Figure 3-8   Reiki self-care position 8.

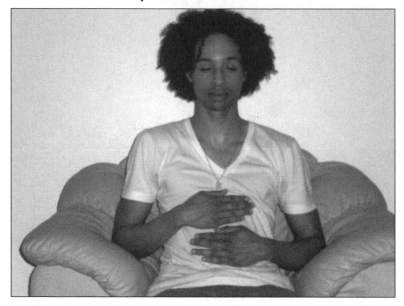

Figure 3-9   Reiki self-care position 9.

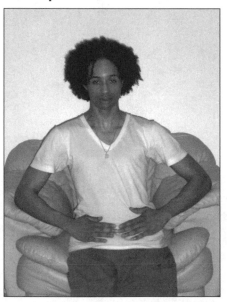

Figure 3-10   Reiki self-care position 10.

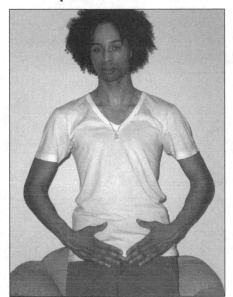

Position #8 (Fig. 3-8): Place both hands on the upper portion of the stomach or middle abdomen.

Position #9 (Fig. 3-9): Place both hands on the lower abdomen or pelvis.

Position #10 (Fig. 3-10): Hold both hands in the center directly above the pubic bone.

Figures 3-11 through 3-14 illustrate the hand placements for the Reiki leg positions.

Position #11 (Fig. 3-11): Hold the front of both knees in way that is comfortable (you can be sitting in a chair).

Position #12 (Fig. 3-12): Hold your right knee and right ankle at the same time (this is done by crossing your leg over your left knee, in a way that is comfortable for you).

Position #13 (Fig. 3-13): Hold your left knee and left ankle at same time (this is done by crossing your leg over your right knee, in a way that is comfortable for you).

Position #14 (Fig. 3-14 a, b): Cradle your right foot with the left and right hands and switch to your left foot with the right and left hands in a way that is the most comfortable for you.

Figure 3-11   Reiki self-care position 11.

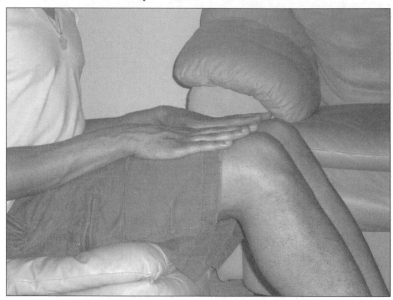

Figure 3-12   Reiki self-care position 12.

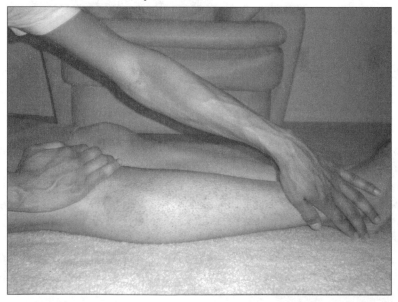

Figure 3-13   Reiki self-care position 13.

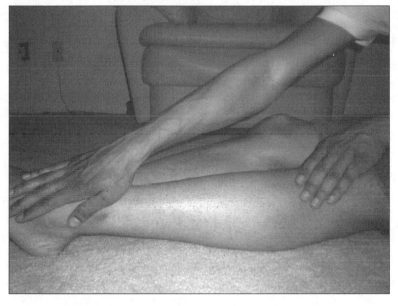

Figure 3-14a   Reiki self-care position 14a.

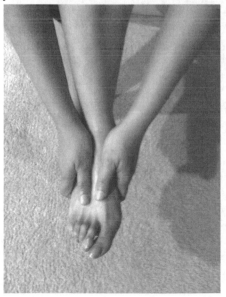

Figure 3-14b   Reiki self-care position 14b.

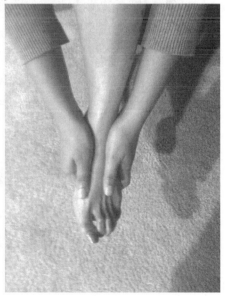

Figures 3-15 through 3-17 illustrate the hand placements for the Reiki back positions.

Position #15 (Fig. 3-15): Place both hands behind you, under your shoulder blades; your fingers should meet mid spine, where the heart is.

Position #16 (Fig. 3-16): Place both hands behind you in the small of your back.

Position #17 (Fig. 3-17): Place both hands behind you in the lower part of your back on your sacrum.

Gently brush yourself off three or four times. Go down the length of your body, sweeping any energetic debris that may have been left over from your self-care session. Remember to drink plenty of water for good health and as part of the cleansing process.

Description of Reiki Self-Care Trading

If you are attuned to Reiki and know other nurses who also practice Reiki, by all means, get together. There is nothing better than meeting another nurse who has been attuned to Reiki. Set up a time to exchange treatments on one another before or after work, or any time when you will not be distracted by work.

Figure 3-15   Reiki self-care position 15.

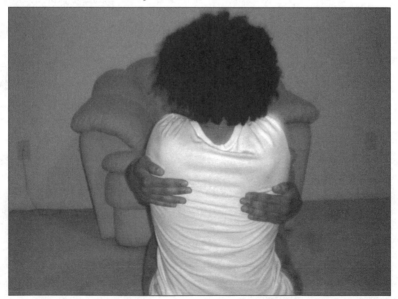

Figure 3-16   Reiki self-care position 16.

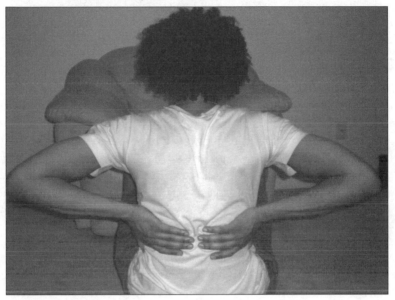

Figure 3-17   Reiki self-care position 17.

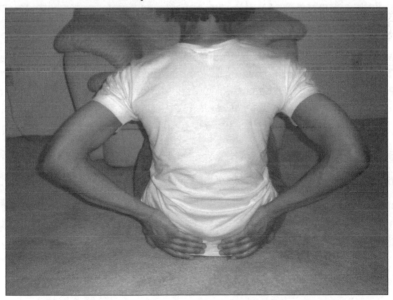

Schedule regular appointments with each other and make a nurturing afternoon out of the Reiki experience. You can talk with other nurses and form classes for further study. This is a benefit to the workplace, the patients, and your families and friends. You can establish loving and compassionate support systems and networks that allow for a community of giving and sharing. When times are hectic, Reiki can help you deal with situations that occur. Nursing takes on a different meaning for everyone, because you are not only licensed to touch and care for others, you also feel destined to touch them. A friendly "heads up": Once people know that you have training and understand the benefits Reiki provides, you will begin to attract many people who are in need of your services. The potential for you to be pretty busy is there. You become a magnet for those in need of healing. This is another good reason to learn self-care. Not only do you care for your families and friends, you care for your patients, caregivers, and coworkers as well. Reiki presents another beautiful opportunity to give to others; however, you must maintain balance.

As a Reiki practitioner the hand positions are similar to the self-care positions, but easier to reach (since you are not performing them on yourself). The session is carried out with the recipient lying on a massage table or sitting in a chair— whatever is comfortable for both participants. Complete the hand positions in the fashion in which you were taught by your teacher, and then switch. The positions have been provided for you in this chapter to refresh your memory, and may vary from what you have been taught in your Reiki classes. Set your intentions and release the worry; there is no wrong way to do Reiki. You have experienced and shared Reiki for your personal self-care. Discuss your experiences with one another and/or record them independently. How are you changing during this time? How do your work environment, relationships, and emotions seem to be changing as you experience Reiki? You may not notice any changes at all, but be observant. Do your hands heat up or cool down at different times during treatment? Do you get images or thoughts about the person you are working on? Share these experiences with your partner or make note of them for further reflection. Schedule the next session and drink plenty of water to keep your body cleansed.

Hand Positions for Reiki Self-Care Trading

Steps:

Imagine that you have a brush or a broom and you are brushing or sweeping completely down your partner's body to begin clearing the clutter from his or her energy field.

Figures 3-18 through 3-21 illustrate the hand placements for the Reiki head position.

Figure 3-18   Reiki self-care trading position 1.

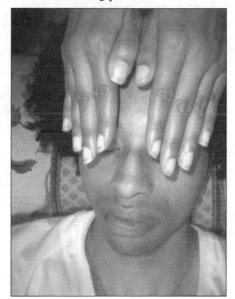

Figure 3-19   Reiki self-care trading position 2.

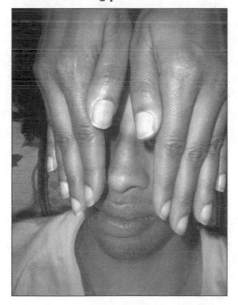

Figure 3-20   Reiki self-care trading position 3.

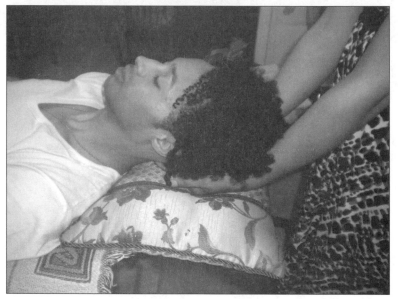

Figure 3-21   Reiki self-care trading position 4.

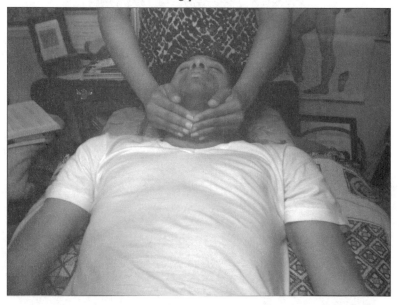

Position #1 (Fig. 3-18): Place your hands over your partner's eyes, gently cupping them.

Position #2 (Fig. 3-19): Cover your partner's cheekbones and temples with your hands, partially covering the ears.

Positions #3 (Fig. 3-20): Gently cradle your partner's head, placing your hands under the back of the head.

Position #4 (Fig. 3-21): Rest both of your hands lightly, with the palms facing your partner's chin, around and over the throat area, resting the sides of the hands where the collarbones meet.

Figures 3-22 through 3-26 illustrate the hand positions for the Reiki trunk positions.

Position #5 (Fig. 3-22): Allow both hands to cover the heart area between the breasts (ask your partner what is most comfortable for him or her).

Position #6 (Fig. 3-23): Place both hands below the breast and slightly above the navel or umbilicus area.

Position #7 (Fig. 3-24): Place both hands beneath the waistline.

Position #8 (Fig. 3-25): Place both hands across the pelvic area right above the pubis.

Figure 3-22   Reiki self-care trading position 5.

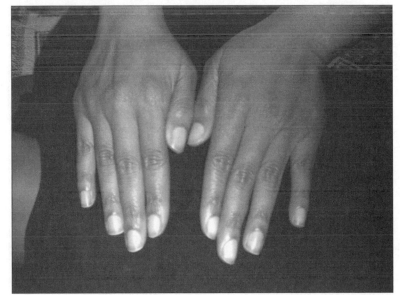

Figure 3-23   Reiki self-care trading position 6.

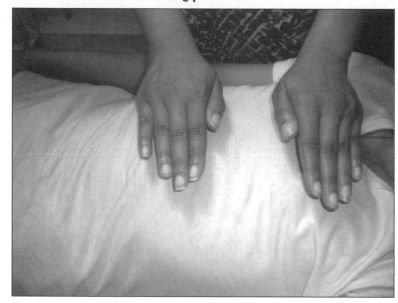

Figure 3-24   Reiki self-care trading position 7.

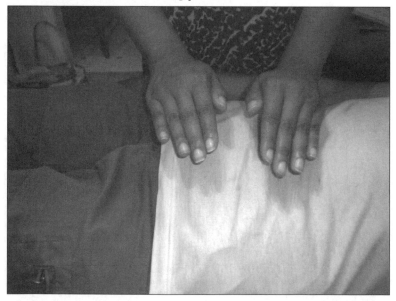

Figure 3-25   Reiki self-care trading position 8.

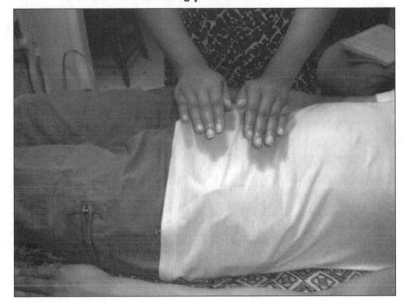

Figure 3-26   Reiki self-care trading position 9.

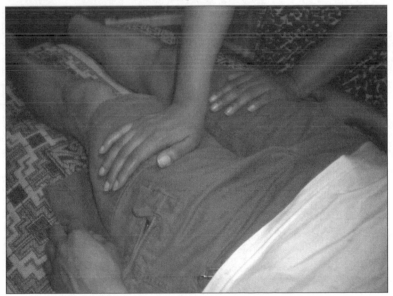

Position #9 (Fig. 3-26): Place both hands midway on the thighs.

Figures 3-27 through 3-31 illustrate the hand positions for the Reiki back positions.

Position #10 (Fig. 3-27): Place your hands horizontally between the upper side of the shoulder and the shoulder blades to the right and left of the spine (back of the neck).

Position #11 (Fig. 3-28): Place your hands horizontally over the shoulder blades (behind the heart chakra).

Position #12 (Fig. 3-29): Place your hands horizontally in the middle of the back.

Position #13 (Fig. 3-30): Place your hands below the waist over the sacral area.

Position #14 (Fig. 3-31): Place your hand over the coccyx.

Figures 3-32 through 3-34 illustrate the hand placements for the Reiki leg positions.

Position #15 (Fig. 3-32): Cover the back of your partner's knees with your hands.

Figure 3-27   Reiki self-care trading position 10.

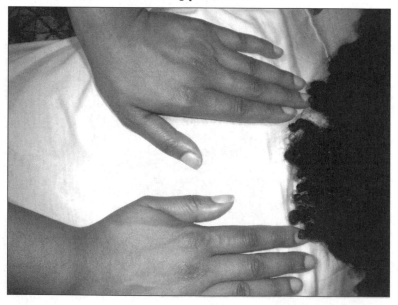

Figure 3-28   Reiki self-care trading position 11.

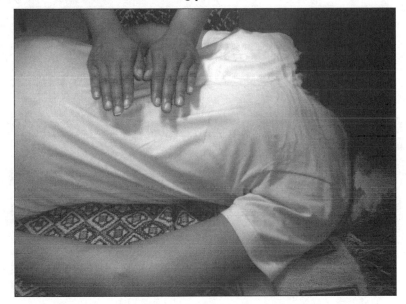

Figure 3-29   Reiki self-care trading position 12.

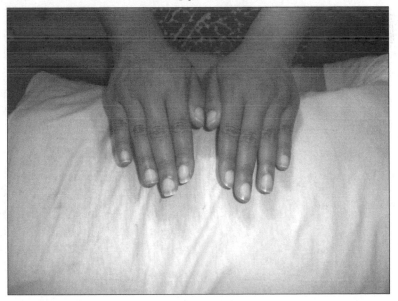

Figure 3-30   Reiki self-care trading position 13.

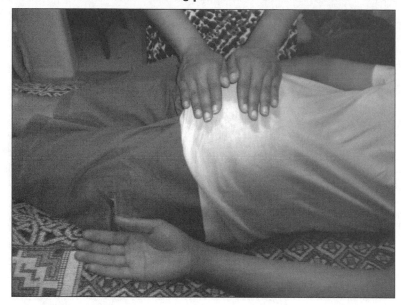

Figure 3-31   Reiki self-care trading position 14.

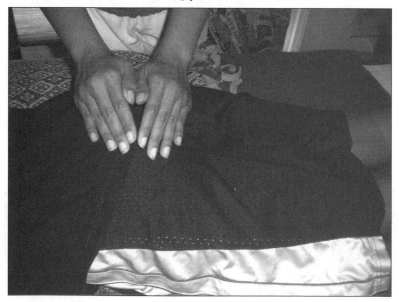

Figure 3-32   Reiki self-care trading position. 15.

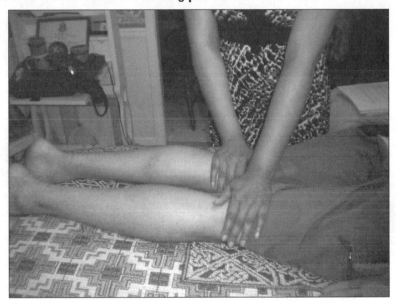

Figure 3-33   Reiki self-care trading position 16.

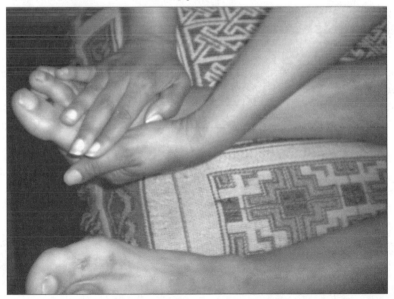

Figure 3-34   Reiki self-care trading position 17.

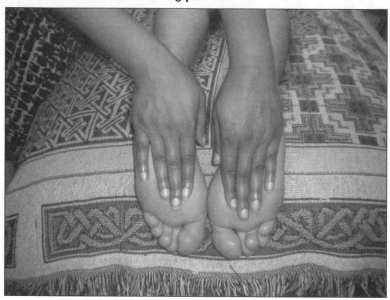

Position #16 (Fig. 3-33): Wrap your hands around your partner's ankles, one at a time.

Position #17 (Fig. 3-34): Place your hands on the soles of your partner's feet, extending from the toes to the middle of the foot; be sure to cover the big toes. This is very grounding.

Gently brush your partner off three or four times. Go down the length of his or her body, sweeping any energetic debris that may have been left over from the self-care session. Remind your fellow nurse to drink plenty of water for good health and as part of the cleansing process.

Benefits of Reiki Self-Care

Benefits on a Physical Level

- Supports immune function
- Increases stamina and endurance
- Energizes the body
- Relaxes stress skeletal and muscular systems
- Reduces and helps alleviate pain
- Can accelerate the healing of wounds and fractures
- Can speed healing of skin (burns, rashes, bruises)

Benefits on Mental and Emotional Levels

- Promotes clarity
- Reduces anxiety
- Promotes stress relief and relaxation.
- Helps with attitudinal and emotional imbalances
- Redistributes energy for overall balance and well-being

Benefits on a Spiritual Level

- Aids interconnectedness with others
- Allows insight into life's purpose
- Helps one experience inner peace and self-love
- Enhances creativity

Further Studies in Usui Reiki

Classes

Classes are offered in many places and can be found by searching listings on holistic or Reiki Web sites, and postings in New Age bookstores. You should select your class carefully, as you would select your Reiki practitioner, doctor, or hair stylist. Meet with members of the class and talk to them about the course, their experiences, and what type of support you will receive from them during this time. During the practice of Reiki, there is a cleansing process that often raises questions in a student's mind (If I'm taking a healing class, why am I sick all of a sudden?). The person may develop symptoms such as feeling tired or weak, or may experience a headache, stomachache, or cold symptoms. It is believed that the body is releasing toxins. The advice is to get more rest during this period, drink plenty of water, and watch your diet. Feel free to discuss this cleansing process with your potential teacher. If he or she is too busy to talk to you, he or she probably is not the right teacher for you.

Usually, four levels of Reiki are taught. Reiki classes are usually conducted over a 2-day period, with Reiki I being taught one day and Reiki II being taught the next. The Reiki Master Class is taught on one day and the Reiki Master Teacher class is taught the next day. Some teachers break the classes up and conduct each one separately over a 2-day period. Many classes are often approved for continuing education hours towards licensure requirements. I would not recommend taking all the classes over a few weekends. Time is needed to process the information, the energy you are feeling, and the changes you might experience once you have been attuned. People sometimes find it hard to believe that they will have this energy for life. Once you have been attuned to Reiki, you never lose the ability to help yourself and others to heal.

Reiki I, or first-degree Reiki (also called Shoden), is taught for the healing of oneself and others. In this class, we focus on healing the self physically and discovering the inner potential we have to be healers in the world. Four initiations are carried out, which provide an attunement to the upper chakras of the body. This prepares one for a future of practicing Reiki on oneself and on others.

Reiki II, or second-degree Reiki (also called Oku Den), focuses on a deeper exploration of self. It enables you to explore personal healing on a physical level, but adds the benefit of allowing you to heal yourself on a mental or emotional level. With the attunement of Reiki II, you can work on yourself and others to help facilitate the healing process.

Reiki III, or third-degree Reiki (also called Shinpiden or mystery teaching) enables you to explore the physical, mental, emotional, and spiritual levels, and bring healing to yourself and others. After Reiki III, a person can choose to teach, and is attuned to the Master symbol. With the final degree of teaching, the student (now teacher) is able to witness the spiritual changes that are occurring in his or her life.

Special Classes

Different classes are offered through various Reiki organizations. William Rand's organization offers advanced Reiki training called Karuna Reiki. This form of Reiki deals with more intense emotional issues and traumas that require support. There are many organizations for Reiki professionals that focus on different topics, such as animal Reiki. See the contact information below to find resources that will help you with your search.

Certification

There are many organizations that have created a certification process for Reiki, but you do not need a certificate to practice or teach Reiki. I have been taught Reiki, but I am not certified by an organization to teach it. I would need a second job if I were formally certified in all the modalities I have been practicing over the years. You do not need any type of credential to teach Reiki, but it is perfect for the nursing profession. Touch is within our scope of practice; therefore, hospitals are becoming open to Reiki being utilized in many capacities.

Contact Information

International Association of Reiki Professionals (IARP)
P.O. Box 104, Harrisville, NH 03450
Phone: 603-881-8838
E-mail: info@iarp.org

International Center for Reiki Training
William Lee Rand
21421 Hilltop St., #28
Southfield, MI 48034
Phone: 248-948-8112, toll free: 800-332-8112
E-mail: center@reiki.org

The Reiki Alliance
Susan Mitchell, Executive Director
Phyllis Lei Furumoto, Grand Master
204 N. Chestnut Street
Kellogg, ID 83837
Phone: 208-783-3535
E-mail: info@reikialliance.c

REFERENCES

Stein, D. (1995). Essential Reiki: *A complete guide to an ancient healing art*. Berkeley, CA: Crossing Press.

Stein, D. (2007). *Essential Reiki teaching manual: A companion guide for teachers*. Berkeley, CA: Crossing Press.

Whelan, K. M. & Wishnia, G. S. (2003). Reiki therapy: The benefits of Reiki to a nurse/Reiki practitioner. *Holistic Nursing Practice*, 17(4), 209–218.

SUGGESTED READING LIST

Brathovde, A. (2006, March-April). A pilot study: Reiki for self-care of nurses and healthcare providers. *Holistic Nursing Practice*, 95–101.

Rand, W. L. (1998). *Reiki for a new millenium*. Southfield, MI: Vision Publications.

Rand, W. L. (2005). *Reiki: The healing touch first and second degree manual*. Southfield, MI: Vision Publications.

Stein, D. (2007). *Essential reiki teaching manual: A companion guide for teachers*. Berkeley, CA: Crossing Press.

Whelan, K. M. (2003). Reiki therapy: The benefits to a nurse/Reiki practitioner. *Holistic Nursing Practice*, 17(4), 209–218.

CHAPTER 4

Introduction to Healing Touch

RACHEL Y. HILL

"Have a heart that never hardens, and a temper that never tires,
and a touch that never hurts."

—CHARLES DICKENS

INTRODUCTION TO HEALING TOUCH

I believe that everything happens for a reason. During the exciting days of completing my master's degree, I was doing a literature search for my research project. I needed to find other modalities to compare with Jin Shin Jyutsu. I knew about Reiki and acupuncture, but I was literally scratching my head trying to figure out what else was out there to compare with Jin Shin Jyutsu. As I was completing my search, I came across information about the Therapeutic Touch and Healing Touch programs. As I read the information more thoroughly, I just sat there in amazement. I was surprised, excited, and pleased all at the same time. I actually went running up and down the halls of the medical center, telling the nurses that Healing Touch was founded by a nurse. Many of my colleagues just shrugged their shoulders matter-of-factly and said they already knew that. A little perturbed, I asked, "Well why didn't anybody bother to tell me, and why isn't anyone taking classes?" Healing Touch was the best-kept secret in town. I didn't know that my fellow nurses were at the forefront of energy medicine. I was excited because I would have more modalities to study in the future. Of course, I was pleased because I finally was able to complete my literature review with the helpful information I had found.

Shortly after I completed my literature search, I looked for a location and took my first class. Each level led to growth and awareness. Level 1, I went to class with a pen and notebook. Level 2, I learned about sharing, because a nurse saw how hungry I was and shared a bag of granola with me. Level 3, I purchased a pendulum that I took very seriously, brought a few snacks for the workshop, and treated myself to a nap during lunchtime. By Level 4, you probably wouldn't have recognized the transformation I had made. I took my own snacks, blankets, pillows, iPod, and anything else that would nurture and pamper me throughout my experience (within reason). It wasn't until I reached Level 4 (which I actually took during the writing of this book) that I gained the truest and deepest sense of what self-care really means. What I appreciate the most about Healing Touch are the role models I have encountered who are living in ways that I can actually envision for myself now. If they can care for themselves, I can too!

History of Healing Touch

Originally known as the Colorado Center for Healing Touch, the Healing Touch Program was born from the experiences and nursing practice of Janet Mentgen. She had been studying energy-based therapies for many years, and exploring the responses patients had to energetic therapies. Janet took specific care to focus on energetic therapies she would use and to note the impact they had on the patient's energy field. She repeatedly experienced great success by using these interventions on patients in her private nursing practice for about 10 years. Janet gathered the techniques she found most beneficial and began to create a more formal structure for energetic practice. Janet Mentgen was definitely not alone in her Healing Touch endeavors, as she was assisted by Shannon Scandrett-Hibdon and Dorothea Hover-Kramer in conducting the first classes in Gainesville, Florida and Memphis, Tennessee. She has also collaborated, taught classes, and coauthored many books with other nurses who are highly recognized in the holistic nursing field. The first four faculty members of the Healing Touch Program were Janet Mentgen, Shannon Scandrett-Hibdon, Dorothea Hover-Kramer, and Myra Till-Tovey (Hover-Kramer, 1996).

In 1990, Healing Touch became a certification program of the American Holistic Nurses Association (AHNA) and a supported program of the American Holistic Medical Association. The AHNA had the resources Janet needed to make Healing Touch a multilevel learning experience for individuals desiring to learn about energy therapy and use it in their own practices. The Healing Touch Program grew tremendously, and eventually, the directors decided it should be separated from the AHNA and become an independent credentialing authority (Healing Touch International, Inc., was formed in 1996). Janet had a great desire for Healing Touch to be recognized as a healing modality that could be covered by insurance companies. She also upheld very high standards of consistency for teaching Healing Touch to practitioners all over the world; therefore, much effort was put into the structuring and credentialing of the program.

The Healing Touch Program went through another change in September of 2005. Janet Mentgen made her peaceful transition from this life, leaving her Healing Touch legacy to her family and her extended Healing Touch family. The Healing Touch Program and Healing Touch International are continuing Janet's vision—meeting the needs of nursing communities, lay communities, and the world. Janet strongly believed that healing should be an opportunity extended to everyone, which is probably the main reason why the program has reached across the world and is shared with many nonnursing practitioners.

Concept of Healing Touch

Healing Touch is a wonderful collection of various energetic healing modalities that have been gathered from various walks of life around the world. Healing Touch allows us to experience the inner power we have to connect with others, balance energy, alleviate discomforts, and facilitate health and well-being. Healing Touch focuses on the various energy fields of the body that have a potential to become disrupted by blockages and stagnation from experience, pain, and trauma. Energy is represented in our bodies by auras, chakras, and meridians. These energetic fields can be detected and help practitioners to sense, see, or feel the disruptions. By using and understanding the different practices learned in Healing Touch, as well as our knowledge of the energy fields of the body, we can help clear the blockages and debris that are causing the imbalances. The modalities used range from meditation to techniques that help to alleviate back ailments, but they all have the specific intent to bring comfort and healing for the highest good. The intention of healing for the highest good basically means that the practitioner desires only what is best for the client to happen at all times. One of the most important concepts in Healing Touch is that Healing Touch practitioners should have a strong awareness of self-care. Nursing and nonnursing practitioners are empowered to nurture themselves in the most divine way possible, just as they nurture others. This creates a balance and makes the treatments more meaningful and effective, because the channels of healing are clear. The receiver and the giver can both experience a moment of mutual connection for the highest good of each other.

Terms Related to Healing Touch

Aura – Metaphysical term for the human energy field, or biofield.

Biofield – A scientific term for the vibrational emanations that surround and extend beyond the human body, as measured by a superconducting quantum interference device (SQUID) and demonstrated through the mechanism of Kirlian photography.

Chakra – Chakra (a Sanskrit word meaning spinning wheel) refers to the human energy centers, or vortices. Chakras are also known as centers of consciousness because of their psychological and developmental properties. The seven major chakras or energy centers are identified by their location, physical area of influence, major psychological function, color, and relationship to the endocrine system. The seven major chakras are the root (or coccygeal), sacral, solar plexus, heart, throat, brow, and crown centers.

Energy blockage – A general term that refers to interruption or constriction of the natural flow patterns in the human vibrational matrix. It may refer to a closed or diminished chakra, asymmetry in the biofield, or nonpolarity and reversal in the meridian flows (Hover-Kramer, 2002).

Human energy system – The human energy system consists of a dynamic interaction of the chakras, the biofield, and the meridians, which together make up the human vibrational matrix of subtle energy (Hover-Kramer, 2002).

Intention – Holding one's inner awareness and focus to accomplish a specific task or activity, being fully present in the moment (Hover-Kramer, 2002).

Meridians – The meridians are the energy tracts of lines of force, though which the life essence travels throughout the entire body. These are used in acupuncture techniques (Hover-Kramer, 2002).

Healing Touch Self-Care Practices

A major emphasis of Janet Mentgen's Healing Touch Program and the Healing Touch organizations is to take care of yourself with the particular care that you would apply to someone else. This isn't an easy feat for caregivers to accomplish. It requires the ability to separate yourself from a role that you are very accustomed to and experience the other end of the spectrum. The Yin-Yang theory comes into play here because we are all givers in our fields of work. We also possess within us the ability to receive, but if we don't allow this natural process to occur, the giving aspect of ourselves will be dominant. The inability to balance our giver and receiver within is where the disharmony comes in. We have to give and receive to keep the flow going. We must learn to give and receive, to and from others and ourselves, in equal proportions.

In 1995, Janet Mentgen gave the keynote address at an AHNA conference. In concluding her remarks, she summarized her rules for tending to the body, mind, and spirit: "We cannot be a spark in someone else's life if our spark has gone out. These are my rules of right rhythmic living. The source of this comes from Alice Bailey and Esoteric Healing. It's been reinforced through me, by my teachers along the path. But this is what I have to do for me on a daily basis" (Mentgen, 2007).

Janet Mentgen's Seven Principles of Self-Care for Healers

1. Physical clearing: Take care of your physical body, your physical existence.
2. Emotional clearing: Express your hurts and pains.
3. Mental clearing: Change your cognitive thought process.
4. Sacred space: Maintain a sacred space at home or away from home.
5. Silence: Practice silent mediation, holy silence.
6. Holy leisure: Restore balance in your life.
7. Holy relationships: Be committed to your relationships.

Self-Care Practice: Experiencing the Seven Principles of Self-Care

Spend some time practicing these principles. Implement each one for a day, a week, or a month to experience the essence of the principle being conveyed to you. The seven principles carry a strong message to nurses about how important it is to revere each other and ourselves in the most special way. Determine what the principles mean to you and design activities to nurture yourself. You may want to create your own set of principles to live and care for yourself by. In doing so, you will begin to notice what is good for yourself and helps you respect what is good for others. You will learn what is not good for yourself or others. You will recognize the reoccurring themes of unrest in your life or experiences that keep coming up that you may not have been willing to face. See how the principles can provide you with a springboard for growth and problem solving. These are various things that can be learning experiences as we apply the seven principles to our lives.

The self-care practices described below have been reinforced in every Healing Touch class I have attended. As a Healing Touch practitioner apprentice, I am even more consistent with maintaining a regular self-care regimen, because of the new things I am learning about energy and our interactions with each other. When I am working with clients, I want my energy to be clear so that I can help them the most. I can sense their imbalances, and they can definitely pick up on my imbalances as well. If I am caring for myself and keeping my energy field balanced, there will be less technical difficulty in the process. I also enjoy the way I feel when I have clarity and feel connected to nature, people, and God. When I feel myself floating away from this point, I do the work that I must do to get me back. The following exercises are priceless for helping you to learn about yourself, balancing your field, and clearing blockages that you might pick up from various interactions in your day.

Chakra Self-Connection

Many Healing Touch techniques use the chakras to harmonize the body. There are many chakras all over our body, although we are most familiar with the seven major ones that align our spinal column. Healing Touch has adapted Brugh Joy's Chakra Connection Technique and utilizes it in the curriculum. This technique can be used as indicated or can be modified for your own personal use. Use this technique upon rising in the morning, during work breaks, and as a quick pick-me-up to keep you going during the day at home or at work.

Benefits
- Connects chakras
- Opens chakras

- Balances the chakras
- Energizes the body

Steps to follow

1. Begin by acknowledging your connection with the supportive universe and sensing your inner center. Set your intention for the help you need.
2. Feeling the energy of the breath in your lungs and heart center gently, let it go to your arms and hands, then connect both hands above and below the foot on the nondominant side.
3. Move your hands higher, connecting the ankle to the knee. Hold until you feel a flow of warmth or a pulsation, a sense of aliveness, moving from the ankle to the knee.
4. Move your hands to connect the knee and hip, holding until you feel the warming flow.
5. Connect in a similar fashion on the dominant side the foot, ankle and knee, and knee and hip.
6. Connect both hips by letting energy flow through the hands to the hips.
7. Connect the root chakra, with one hand below or on the perineum and the other on the sacral center, just below the umbilicus.
8. When you feel a flow of vitality from the feet through the lower abdomen, move higher by placing one hand on the sacral center and the other on the solar plexus. You will know exactly how much holding you need in this vulnerable area to recharge your batteries and to feel genuinely nurtured.
9. Feeling the support of all the lower centers, connect the solar plexus and heart center by sensing the flow of unconditional love toward others and yourself.
10. With one hand on your heart, let the other hand connect to the wrist, elbow, and shoulder. Alternate so that the other hand is on the heart center and you connect the other wrist, elbow, and shoulder.
11. Place both hands on both shoulders, giving yourself a nice big hug. Remember that all we do for ourselves is an extension of the gifts of universal love, of which there is a limitless supply.
12. Connect the heart chakra and the throat center, the throat and the brow, and the brow and the crown. Finally, connect the crown and the transpersonal point above the crown to celebrate your connection with a higher power as you understand it. Feel the boundaries of your marvelous energy being that extends out about as far as your hands can reach. And now, you are ready for whatever is next on your agenda (Hover-Kramer, 2002).

Figure 4-1 illustrates another self-help practice called the "self-full-body connection." It is similar to the chakra connection and involves a few more steps, as described below.

Figure 4-1   Self full body connection.

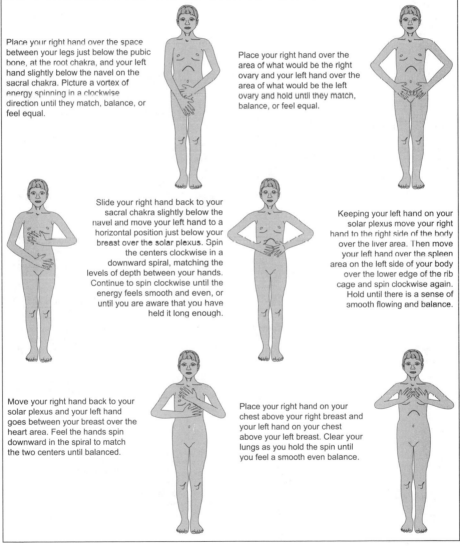

Place your right hand over the space between your legs just below the pubic bone, at the root chakra, and your left hand slightly below the navel on the sacral chakra. Picture a vortex of energy spinning in a clockwise direction until they match, balance, or feel equal.

Place your right hand over the area of what would be the right ovary and your left hand over the area of what would be the left ovary and hold until they match, balance, or feel equal.

Slide your right hand back to your sacral chakra slightly below the navel and move your left hand to a horizontal position just below your breast over the solar plexus. Spin the centers clockwise in a downward spiral, matching the levels of depth between your hands. Continue to spin clockwise until the energy feels smooth and even, or until you are aware that you have held it long enough.

Keeping your left hand on your solar plexus move your right hand to the right side of the body over the liver area. Then move your left hand over the spleen area on the left side of your body over the lower edge of the rib cage and spin clockwise again. Hold until there is a sense of smooth flowing and balance.

Move your right hand back to your solar plexus and your left hand goes between your breast over the heart area. Feel the hands spin downward in the spiral to match the two centers until balanced.

Place your right hand on your chest above your right breast and your left hand on your chest above your left breast. Clear your lungs as you hold the spin until you feel a smooth even balance.

(continued)

Figure 4-1   *(continued)*

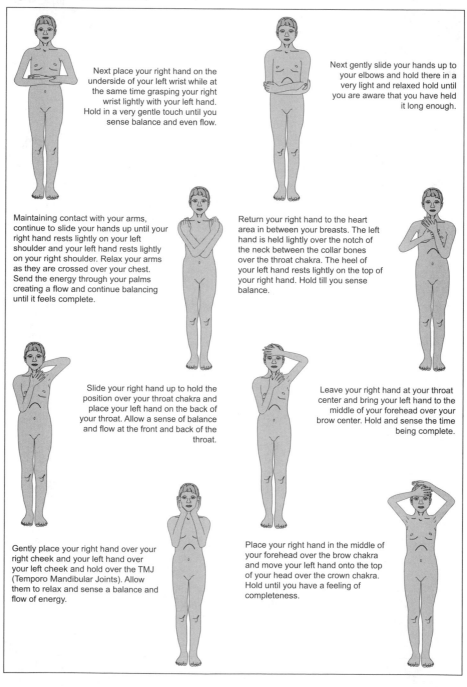

Next place your right hand on the underside of your left wrist while at the same time grasping your right wrist lightly with your left hand. Hold in a very gentle touch until you sense balance and even flow.

Next gently slide your hands up to your elbows and hold there in a very light and relaxed hold until you are aware that you have held it long enough.

Maintaining contact with your arms, continue to slide your hands up until your right hand rests lightly on your left shoulder and your left hand rests lightly on your right shoulder. Relax your arms as they are crossed over your chest. Send the energy through your palms creating a flow and continue balancing until it feels complete.

Return your right hand to the heart area in between your breasts. The left hand is held lightly over the notch of the neck between the collar bones over the throat chakra. The heel of your left hand rests lightly on the top of your right hand. Hold till you sense balance.

Slide your right hand up to hold the position over your throat chakra and place your left hand on the back of your throat. Allow a sense of balance and flow at the front and back of the throat.

Leave your right hand at your throat center and bring your left hand to the middle of your forehead over your brow center. Hold and sense the time being complete.

Gently place your right hand over your right cheek and your left hand over your left cheek and hold over the TMJ (Temporo Mandibular Joints). Allow them to relax and sense a balance and flow of energy.

Place your right hand in the middle of your forehead over the brow chakra and move your left hand onto the top of your head over the crown chakra. Hold until you have a feeling of completeness.

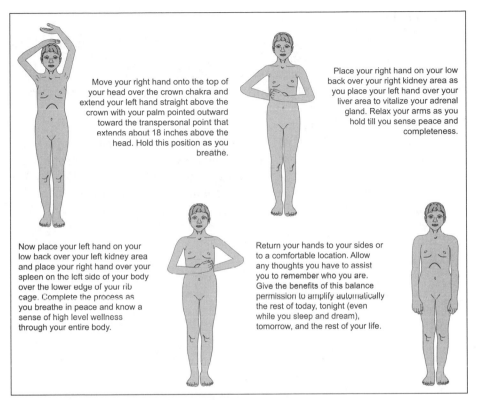

Move your right hand onto the top of your head over the crown chakra and extend your left hand straight above the crown with your palm pointed outward toward the transpersonal point that extends about 18 inches above the head. Hold this position as you breathe.

Place your right hand on your low back over your right kidney area as you place your left hand over your liver area to vitalize your adrenal gland. Relax your arms as you hold till you sense peace and completeness.

Now place your left hand on your low back over your left kidney area and place your right hand over your spleen on the left side of your body over the lower edge of your rib cage. Complete the process as you breathe in peace and know a sense of high level wellness through your entire body.

Return your hands to your sides or to a comfortable location. Allow any thoughts you have to assist you to remember who you are. Give the benefits of this balance permission to amplify automatically the rest of today, tonight (even while you sleep and dream), tomorrow, and the rest of your life.

Courtesy of Debra Basham and Joel P. Bowman–SCS Matters, LLC

Chakra Meditation

The chakra meditation is a meditation that does not require you to be totally still. There is the movement of the hand from one chakra to the next, which helps to stimulate the chakra energy and increase the effects of each chakra. This meditation can be done in the morning to begin the day. It can also be done at the end of the day, when you might be experiencing fatigue. It can be performed at work on breaks, and used when you're feeling disappointed or discouraged. Once the chakras are stimulated, you will be able to reconnect to the universal life force and recognize where the true power in the situation lies.

Benefits

- Provides balance and harmony
- Allows one to sense one's true power and connectedness
- Revitalizes and replenishes physically, mentally, and spiritually

Steps to follow

1. Set your intention for the healing you wish for yourself. Begin to mobilize the healing forces within by identifying what you want to heal or release.
2. Begin with the spine in alignment, either lying down or sitting up in a comfortable position. Celebrate your aliveness with a positive statement such as, I feel my joy; vitality is now flowing through me; I deserve love and now attract loving thoughts.
3. Releasing any tension with the out-breath, allow your hands to move to the root chakra area...feel your life force, your sense of belonging on the Earth, your sense of safety and security with yourself. Hold each position for 1 to 3 minutes depending on your sense of what is needed for each area.
4. Move both hands to the sacral chakra...sense your body in balance; sense your emotional nature, and make note of any current feeling for later attention, and release what is not needed at this time.
5. Move your hands over the solar plexus area....notice how good it feels to protect that vulnerable area. Allow yourself to take in energy from the universe in the form of golden sunlight, wind, or ocean waves...sense your ability to be assertive and effective in communicating with others.
6. Move both hands to the heart center...feel the flow of unconditional love toward others; feel their love flowing into you. Send out the flow of this love to yourself, forgiving easily and learning from all past experiences. Feel the support of the three lower centers as you do this.
7. Move the hands to the throat center...sense your ability to express your being; enjoy singing, chanting, making sounds, speaking with clarity.
8. Proceed to the brow center, the intuitive chakra....sense your awareness expanding, and the ability to see with insight and wisdom. See all there is to see; sense what another person's situation might be. Allow yourself an insight about the current situation.
9. Reach to the crown chakra, feeling your connection with the infinite...unlimited resources of love and wisdom are available to you through this connection.
10. Slowly relax the hands, continuing to feel your energy flow as you move forward and set your intent for the next activity of the day (Hover-Kramer, 1996).

Heart-Centering Meditation

Self-care always begins with a centering of the self to create the highest good for oneself. This process allows you to attain inner peace and stillness to focus on your individual needs. Heart-centering meditation can be practiced two or three times daily, for periods of 15 to 20 minutes. It is perfect for morning, lunch, and afternoon breaks. Practice this centering until it becomes an automatic response, allowing you to go within in times of difficulty and emerge as your true self.

Benefits

- Inner peace
- Self-awareness
- Improved attitude and coping ability
- Balance
- Unconditional love
- Stress relief
- Focus
- Clarity

Steps to follow

1. Allow your awareness to move to your heart center...take a slow, deep breath and feel the energy.
2. Visualize an emerald green light at the heart center...feel the sensation of warmth and balance move into your chest, shoulders, arms, head, abdomen, thighs, legs, and feet...relax the entire body. If the mind wanders, refocus at the heart center and repeat the process.
3. See with your inner eye a friend or someone you wish to help. Sense your heart center opening to the person in front of you and note how good it feels to send out the vibration of caring.
4. Allow the person in front of you to be yourself, perhaps as a little child, or at a time that was difficult or when you were embarrassed about something.
5. Allow that same quality of love and compassion you had for your friend to go to yourself. Forgive and feel the vibration of compassion. Allow yourself to learn from the difficult experience. Be very gentle with yourself.
6. Connect again with the breath and gently come back to full awareness (Hover-Kramer, 2002).

Community Healing Touch Meetings

There are many areas with thriving Healing Touch communities. Check with the various Healing Touch organizations to find out what events and activities are currently taking place in your city. There may be monthly meetings in which practitioners, practitioner-apprentices (who have the wonderful opportunity to give 100 free sessions to complete their certification), and Healing Touch students at other levels get together and share treatments with one another. The Healing Touch networks offer their healing services to many different camps during the summer. They spend a great deal to provide care to cancer patients and survivors, children with special needs, and staff and patients at hospice houses. This is an excellent opportunity to learn more about Healing Touch and experience sessions for yourself, and learn ways to keep yourself healthy.

Experiencing Healing Touch as a Client

Selecting a practitioner

Private sessions are another option for self-care. You can select a practitioner by word of mouth or searching the phone book or New Age newspapers and magazines (be sure to ask about the practitioner's credentials). However, I always recommend searching in the directory listings maintained by Healing Touch organizations. I suggest these sources first, because individuals on their lists have met the recommendations of the Healing Touch organizations. Because not every practitioner will be listed, however, you should always ask about certifications and confirm with both organizations if there is any question.

Pricing for sessions

Pricing for sessions ranges from $65 to $85, which is similar to pricing for massages and other holistic modalities.

Duration and frequency of sessions

Sessions range from 45 minutes to 1.5 hours. The frequency of the session depends on the condition of the client. Clients who are severely ill can only tolerate small amounts of therapy at a time. Usually, animals and children will get what they need from you and decide when they are done. The number of sessions also depends on what needs to be accomplished. It is a mutual decision made by you and your practitioner.

What to expect from a session

A medical history is usually gathered before the session begins. A quick intake can sometimes be taken over the phone and completed more fully in person. The practitioner will ask questions pertaining to your experience with energy work, medications, pain issues you might be experiencing, your current pain level, and any device you might be wearing that regulates your body functions in some way (such as a pacemaker, pain pump, or insulin pump). The practitioner will also ask what your health concerns are, and the main reason for your seeking treatment. If you are unfamiliar with energy work, the practitioner will educate you about the methods used and provide information about what you will experience in a session. The two of you will decide as a team on a mutual goal for the outcome of your session, and begin to visualize the outcome you both desire. The practitioner will determine, based on your intake and medical history, what techniques will be best for you. This is determined by intuition as well as by knowledge about your health challenge and what has worked in the past. The practitioner will explain the plan and techniques that will be used, and you will be invited to rest on the table and receive the treatment. The session begins usually with the practitioner doing a self-centering or grounding of himself or herself to create an environment within that promotes healing and peace. This centering includes prayer, setting the intention, and honoring your presence as an opportunity to grow. The practitioner will then assess your energy field, using a pendulum held a few inches over each of the seven main energy centers (chakras), or by running his or her hand slowly down your energy field a few inches off the body. The practitioner will be able to "get a feel" for what might be occurring with you energetically. Healing Touch is not a massage, but people seem to rest quickly and easily once a session begins. The relaxed state allows the body to begin its healing process. The practitioner will be attentive throughout the session so that any necessary changes in technique will be detected and implemented for your benefit. The practitioner will "ground" you at the end of the session to help bring you to the here and now. You will become fully alert, but will be allowed to rest on the table until you have regained your bearings. Get assistance from the practitioner before you attempt to get off the table. Once you are fully present, the practitioner will review the session with you, exchange feedback about the session, and discuss follow-up measures and self-care (you decide upon) for your maintenance and personal growth. The practitioner will offer you water so that you can begin flushing your systems of impurities, and because it is just plain good for you.

Further Studies in Healing Touch

Classes

Healing Touch is a multilevel program for nurses (and non-nurses) to explore energy-based modalities that have been gathered from various healing traditions locally and all around the world. The courses range from Level 1 for beginners to Level 6 for those desiring to teach Healing Touch to others. A number of advanced training and recognition courses of energetic therapy teach many techniques that can be used to help bring comfort and balance in various settings and conditions of illness and disease. Continuing education is granted for nurses who participate, based on the time spent in each workshop. Two Healing Touch training programs are available to those who wish to study Healing Touch. Healing Touch International is the path I chose, because the classes were offered in my local area. However, the training programs of Healing Touch International and the Healing Touch Program are similar. If you choose to study further, you are free to explore which path is right for you.

Level 1

Level 1 is the introductory-level workshop and is open to all persons regardless of their background and training. The workshop is usually 2 days long and is usually conducted over a weekend. In Level 1, many energetic concepts are discussed. The human energy field is described as it relates to modern scientific principles. The instructor will have had a great deal of experience with Healing Touch, and will be able to share that experience and feedback with the students. Students will have the opportunity to explore and experience the principles of Healing Touch, and to demonstrate the sequence of each step in the various healing techniques that are discussed during the workshop. Level 1 students will also be taught when it is most appropriate to use certain Healing Touch interventions, and how to apply these specific interventions to themselves and others.

Level 2

Before you can take a Level 2 workshop, you must have completed the Level 1 workshop. This workshop is also usually completed over 2 days (usually a weekend). Level 2 exposes the student to a deeper level of theory, knowledge, and practice. This course teaches several additional healing techniques that allow you to move toward being an advanced practitioner, and to treat clients with specific mental, neck, and back discomforts. During this course, students learn the techniques and become comfortable in demonstrating them, while they also continue to develop their ability to use instruments for assessment, such as the pendulum and the hand. The students learn what is involved in an hour-long session with a client, and are given the opportunity to utilize all they have learned thus far.

Level 3

The Level 2 workshop is a prerequisite for the Level 3 workshop. The knowledge base delves deeper into concepts that relate to "supernatural realms." Students learn about the higher sensory perception and the innate ability we possess to use our intuition or the highest part of our consciousness to help others to heal. More advanced healing techniques are taught, learned, and practiced that enable the students to prepare for working with the higher vibrational energy levels. Self-care and the self-development of the healer are topics that are thoroughly discussed to support the student in his or her advancement as a healer. Assigned readings help the students expand their knowledge about the human energy system and the use of tools, and to skillfully integrate the advanced techniques into a full healing sequence for a client.

Level 4

Level 4 is for students who have completed Levels 1, 2, and 3. This level is more on the order of a retreat and is reserved for those who want to become practitioners and receive certification in Healing Touch. In Level 4, students review all of the techniques of Healing Touch, and become proficient in articulating the uses of each technique and when to apply them. Students learn the ethics of Healing Touch, as well as how to begin a professional practice as a Healing Touch practitioner. Upon completion of the Level 4 Healing Touch class, the student becomes a Healing Touch student/apprentice. A certified Healing Touch practitioner is assigned to each Level 4 student as a mentor to assist, coach, support, and guide the student toward successful completion of the certification requirements.

Level 5 and Certification

Level 4 is a prerequisite for Level 5. Level 4 focuses on the business concepts, ethics, appropriate relationships between the client and the therapist, and various ways to create community healthcare programs. When a student completes the requirements for Level 4, he or she is ready for Level 5. The Healing Touch mentor interacts with the student, experiencing the Healing Touch techniques as applied by the student. The student is required to complete 100 documented sessions with clients and a specific number of case studies, and read certain books, among other things. The number of sessions allows students to increase their knowledge about the energetic techniques they are learning, so that they can demonstrate a superior understanding of the concepts and energetic healing principles. The student/apprentice is required to receive 12 treatments from other complementary modalities outside of Healing Touch. As the practitioner is giving sessions to meet requirements, this ensures that the practitioner is receiving other treatments to enrich his or her own self-care experience. To become a Certified Healing Touch Practitioner the necessary requirements are submitted, case studies are presented orally during the Level 5 workshop, a personal portfolio is created of the practitioner-apprentice's accomplishments and healing touch experience, and the remaining paperwork requirements are mailed into the Healing Touch International Headquarters for review. The student/apprentices and mentors patiently wait to hear from the certification board regarding acceptance of the application.

Level 6

In Level 6, students receive training that allows them to teach Healing Touch to others. Certified practitioners can participate if they choose to expand their experience to that of teacher. The core emphasis for the group is to discuss dynamics, different styles of learning, methods of teaching others, and the creation of programs. Those who become instructors meet together yearly to further their studies, advance their skills, brainstorm about new and innovative possibilities for Healing Touch, and network.

The Healing Touch International and Healing Touch Program Web sites contain more specific details about the requirements for the different levels of training, tuition costs for each class, locations, dates, and times for each upcoming class. The Web sites are listed in the contact information.

Special Classes

Special classes are often given that can be very useful in helping you practice self-care to a greater extent. They can help empower you and create networks of support. Take advantage of the workshops that are offered as part of your growth. A Healing Touch for Self-Care class is taught in conjunction with the Healing Touch Program. This class was envisioned, created, and taught by Barbara Ann Starke, RN, MSN, FNP, AHN-BC, CHTP/I, NADA Trainer, who once wrote, "There is a power in taking care of the Light within me so I may help your Light shine (Starke, 2008). This class and other special topic classes are periodically taught and are usually 1 or 2 days long. Other specialty classes cover many topics, ranging from anatomy reviews to Healing Touch for animals. Check the various Healing Touch Web sites and get on their mailing lists so that you can be notified when the classes are available. Some classes may require the completion of a certain level, but you can check the registration information and get clarification if needed.

Additional Resources

The Healing Touch Program produces a monthly magazine called *Energy Magazine*. This magazine is available to you by e-mail; simply go to the Web site and subscribe. The magazine contains articles by practitioners and educational information that can further your knowledge about energy work, working with patients, and self-care.

Contact Information

Healing Touch International, Inc.
445 Union Blvd., Suite 105
Lakewood, CO 80228
Phone: 303-989-7982
Fax: 303-980-8683
http://www.healingtouchinternational.org
Healing Touch Program
San Antonio Office
20822 Cactus Loop
San Antonio, TX 78258

Phone: 210-497-5529
Fax: 210-497-8532
Denver Office
5783 Sheridan Blvd., Suite 101
Arvada, CO 80002
Phone: 303-989-0581
Fax: 303-985-9702
Office hours: 9:00 a.m. to 5:00 p.m. weekdays (answering machine on after hours).
E-mail: info@HealingTouchProgram.com
http://www.HealingTouchProgram.com

Healing Touch Professional Association (HTPA)
(Membership association, in conjunction with the Healing Touch Program, for practitioners who practice Healing Touch)
20822 Cactus Loop, Suite 300
San Antonio, TX 78258
Phone: 210-497-5529
Fax: 210-497-8532
E-mail: info@HTProfessionalAssociation.com

HT Worldwide Foundation, Inc.
(Nonprofit organization to help spread Healing Touch globally)
16211 Clay Road, Suite 106, Box 215
Houston, TX 77084
Phone: 281-856-8340
E-mail: HTWFoundation@aol.com

REFERENCES

Hover-Kramer, D. (1996). *Healing Touch: A resource for health care professionals.* Albany, NY: Delmar Publishers.

Hover-Kramer, D. (2002). *Healing Touch: A guidebook for practitioners.* Albany, NY: Delmar Publishing.

Mentgen, J. (2007). Path of healership: The importance of self care for the healer. *Energy Magazine*, July. pp. 15–18.

Starke, B. A. (2008). Healing Touch for self-care. *Energy Magazine*, March. pp. 14–16.

SUGGESTED READING LIST

Healing Touch Program's – Energy Magazine – Monthly publication
Healing Touch International's Perspectives in Healing – Quarterly publication

CHAPTER 5

Introduction to Hypnosis

RACHEL Y. HILL

*"The greatest discovery of this generation is that
human beings can alter their lives by altering their attitude of mind."*
—ALBERT SCHWEITZER

INTRODUCTION TO HYPNOSIS

We are able to accomplish so many things when we put our mind to it. Even when the resources are not always available to accomplish a specific task, the mind has a way of compensating for the deficit and revealing creative ways to overcome the dilemma. Imagine a little baby who is discovering how to crawl. The baby sees something fascinating in a room and begins to make their way to that object, despite their novice crawling abilities. The baby might waddle, roll, slide, and scoot with highly focused attention. Before we know it, he or she has arrived at the object of interest. Nurses are faced with challenges daily. Unfortunately, at times there can be a lack of resources, lack of support, and lack of morale in the workplace. These trying times can create feelings of hopelessness and helplessness and a lack of motivation to accomplish the tasks required for general patient care. How do we overcome the hardship, create the best outcome for the patient, and reestablish balance in the workplace and within ourselves?

The key to overcoming hardship is to overcome the limitations that overshadow the solutions. Limitations can come from outside you, from people, physical conditions, bureaucracies, etc. Other limitations can come from within you, such as self-esteem issues, negative thinking, doubt, fear, etc. Being successful means overcoming all limitations, and this usually starts with your mind. Hypnosis or hypnotherapy is one way you can bring your conscious mind and your subconscious mind together to achieve things that you desire or need. As the slogan goes, the mind is a terrible thing to waste—and I couldn't agree more. The mind is a very powerful tool that can help us overcome challenges and maintain a healthy balance in our lives. Hypnosis is not just for problems or challenges. Hypnosis can be used to achieve radiance, deeper understanding, memory enhancement, connections with the highest true self, and many other possibilities. However, without the agreement of your minds (subconscious and conscious), it will be difficult to achieve the things in life you desire.

History of Hypnosis

- The Sumerians practiced hypnosis 4000 years before the time of Christ, as described on cuneiform tablets. The priest of Erech had a manuscript that supposedly proved that cures had been achieved through hypnotic suggestions. The Sumerians believed there were three grades of hypnotherapy: light hypnosis, medium hypnosis, and deep hypnosis.
- The Law of Manu, the ancient science of India, defines the levels of hypnosis as the sleep-waking state, the dream-sleep, and the ecstasy-sleep. The Ebers papyrus, found in Egypt, shows many methods of hypnosis that were used as a therapy tool. Priests were regarded as doctors in ancient Egypt, and they used the power of suggestion. Patients would stare at metal discs, which created a fatigue that would cause them to fall into a hypnotic sleep. This technique came to be known as "fixation" and is commonly used in hypnosis today.
- In Greece, sleep temples were used. Individuals who were seeking healing followed special diets, took special baths, and participated in special cleansing rituals. The priest told them about cures that helped others in their condition, which encouraged them mentally and stimulated their expectations for the same healing to occur with them.
- In ancient Rome, doctors served as middlemen between the gods and the ill. Certain philosophers also began to use the power of suggestion that was used by physicians.
- Many of the healing techniques documented in the Old and New Testaments in the Bible have been linked to hypnosis. Ansari (1991) noted that, "In pre-Christian times, the Jews used professional exorcists. These practices cannot be described as anything but what we know today as hypnosis."
- In the second century A.D., a poet named Porphyrus reported an argument between two students, Plotinus and Olympius, over the beliefs of their masters regarding hypnosis. To settle the disagreement, Olympius challenged Plotinus to prove his gift in the art of hypnosis. People gathered around and watched attentively. Plotinus stared at Olympius for a few minutes, probably in an intimidating way, and called out, "Behold, his body shrivels like a purse!" Olympius received the suggestion mentally, felt a great pain shoot through his body, and agreed that the mental strength of Plotinus was far superior to his own.
- Paracelsus (1493–1541) is famous for saying, "The deciding factor in a cure is the inner doctor." He was at risk of being executed because of the various treatments he used (hypnosis being one of them), which were considered satanic.
- Maximilian Hell (1720–1792) was a famous astronomer and Jesuit priest who achieved cures through the use of magnets. He would place magnets on images of diseased organs or places where pain existed in the body, and 60% to 80% improvement in his patients' physical condition.

- Friedrick Anton Mesmer (1734–1815) is considered the father of modern hypnosis. The term "mesmerize" stems from his name. He believed that he could cure sick people by magnetizing their fluids. This was achieved by passing a hand along the length of the patient's body, from the top of the head to the soles of the feet. This would cause a convulsing effect, and the patient would then fall into a deep sleep. Louis XVI commissioned the Royal Academy of Sciences to examine Mesmer's doctrines. He was discredited, ridiculed, and called a quack by the commission. The patients' convulsions were considered immoral, despite the healing impact afterward. Mesmer died discouraged and in poverty.
- James Braid (1795–1860) was an English ophthalmologist who observed experiments conducted by LaFontaine, a magnetist. He studied these experiments to disprove the theory of hypnosis. After practicing the techniques on his wife, friend, and servant, however, he was able to make them fall asleep by staring at a button on the tip of his nose. It was Braid who coined the term "hypnosis."
- Sigmund Freud is the founder of psychoanalysis. He confirmed the occurrence of hypnosis, but was unable to perform it successfully on his clients and therefore discouraged the use of it.
- Émile Coué developed the doctrine of self-hypnosis or auto suggestion. He believed any individual can be a powerful hypnotherapist. He also proposed three laws of hypnotherapy: (1) the law of concentrated attention, (2) the law of dominant effect, and (3) the law of dominant action.
- Jean Martin Charcot (1825–1893) was a neurologist who worked with many illnesses and revolutionized hypnotherapy. He used a "shock technique" to startle groups of people and cause them to fall into a hypnotic state.
- I. P. Pavlov believed that hypnosis and the power of suggestion are phenomena that are inherent in daily life.
- The British Medical Association approved the study of hypnosis in medical schools and postgraduate curricula, and approved its use for psychiatric and surgical purposes.
- The American Medical Association followed suit and integrated hypnosis into its curricula.
- Doctors in World War I and World War II used hypnosis to treat neuroses. During the Korean War, hypnotherapy and psychology became connected together (Ansari, 1991).

Concept of Hypnosis

We use only a small capacity of our brain compared with what we have available. Hypnosis is a tool that allows us to explore the unused potential of our minds to accomplish the goals we desire. Hypnosis is a significant tool commonly used in complementary therapy practices today. Psychologists, surgeons, dentists, and other healthcare practitioners are finding the benefits of hypnosis to be very useful in their settings. With this technique, the hypnotherapist takes you to a certain point of relaxation, called the alpha state. In this state you are the most receptive of suggestions for change. Suggestions are given to you in this state, your mind receives them, and you have new patterns for change that have been downloaded to your mind (like software for a new computer). When the session is over, you experience changes that help you to see and experience what your mind is able to do with a little restructuring, help, and determination to change. Hypnosis is beneficial for changing behaviors and thought patterns, alleviating pain, overcoming challenges, achieving wellness, and many more things. Exploring hypnosis is very important because we are allowing our brains to be used in a wider capacity, creating new brain pathways and tapping into our hidden potential. Understanding the way the mind works, knowing what to feed your mind, and getting your two minds (the conscious and subconscious) to work together are important parts of successful hypnosis. The conscious mind is the part of our brain that makes plans, decisions, and controls our day-to-day activities. The conscious mind stops functioning when we are asleep. When the conscious mind shuts down, the subconscious mind takes over and protects the body by regulating the heart, body temperature, and respiratory systems. The subconscious mind is always functioning and never takes a break. An example of how the subconscious mind protects you is when you have driven home, but don't remember driving. When you first learned how to drive, it was a conscious act. Once you have driven thousands of times, your subconscious mind can come to your rescue (on one of those days after a long shift when you are very tired and can barely keep your eyes open). Once you arrive home safely, you may not remember driving home, but it feels almost like you have "driven in your sleep" because another part of your mind was engaged. This expression characterizes the many things we do that become embedded in our subconscious mind after time; they are conscious activities, but at the same time can be carried out subconsciously too. When you daydream, dream at night, or have experiences that take you out of your normal conscious state, you are engaging your subconscious mind.

The conscious mind analyzes what is possible and what isn't. The subconscious mind knows no bounds and has all your habits committed to memory. Therefore, when you want to lose weight, because you "consciously" know it is good for you, you must also work with the subconscious mind to make this happen. Your subconscious mind must relearn old eating habits you have established and be constantly reminded of what you want to accomplish, as opposed to what you have not. When a child is in danger and pinned under a car, his mother may be able to find the ability to pick the car up and save her child. She doesn't think about the car being so heavy. She thinks about the life of her child. The mother bypasses the conscious mind that would analyze the weight of the car and say such a thing would be impossible. She is aware of the direct need to save her child, and therefore lifting the car is the only option. The subconscious mind agrees and allows it to happen.

In relating hypnosis to the work setting and personal need for self-care, the possibilities are endless. Any issue you face with coworkers, patients, or yourself can be dealt with by hypnotherapy.

Terms Related to Hypnosis

Alpha state – The state in which we are receptive of suggestions during hypnosis. We are so relaxed that we can hear the phone ring, but we don't move and stay in our relaxed state.

Beta state – The state that describes our waking consciousness (e.g., going to work, having conversations, or planning the menu for dinner).

Delta state – The state of deep sleep.

Autohypnosis – Hypnotizing yourself.

Conscious mind – The part of your mind that makes decisions and is awake during the day.

Ego – The part of your consciousness that wants to control and protect you and the way you have always been during your life.

Hypnotherapist – A licensed professional who has been trained to hypnotize others.

Hypnosis – The art of getting a person's subconscious mind and conscious mind to work together for a common good and achieve what a desired goal.

Hypnotist – A nonlicensed individual who has been trained to hypnotize others.

Law of concentrated attention – An idea tends to realize itself when we focus our attention on it.

Law of dominant effect – Accompanying a suggestion with a strong emotion enhances the suggestion. Any prior suggestion is replaced by the combination of the emotion-suggestion.

Law of reverse action – The harder you try to accomplish a task, the more difficult it is to achieve.

Theta state – A slower state than the alpha state; in this state we can do things automatically, but not consciously (e.g., forgetting what we just did within the past 3 minutes, driving and not remembering the ride home).

Trance – A state of altered consciousness in which an individual is relaxed and not totally connected to his or her present physical surroundings.

Subconscious mind – The part of the mind that maintains bodily functions while we sleep, and goes out and about while we are dreaming.

Myths (and Truths) about Hypnosis

- Your give control of your mind to someone else. (You are always in control.)
- You are asleep and unaware of your surroundings. (You are awake and more sensitive to your surroundings, and your senses are heightened.)
- You will reveal all of your deep dark secrets to others. (You will not tell secrets that you have no desire to share, because you are in control.)
- Suggestions won't be remembered after the session. (You will remember the suggestions and hypnosis experience once it is over.)
- You will pick up another bad habit to replace the one you have gotten rid of. (You won't accept anything you don't want to accept. As long as the cause of an issue has been removed, you won't accept another unwanted habit.)
- You will be stuck in hypnosis. (You will come out of hypnosis when you are ready to.)

Facts about Hypnosis

- The subject will not do anything contrary to his or her moral principles.
- Hypnosis is not a sleep state; awareness is increased.
- You do not have to be in a deep state for hypnosis to benefit you.
- The more intelligent and imaginative the subject is, the easier it will be to hypnotize him or her.
- The subject remains aware of everything that is going on.

HYPNOSIS SELF-CARE PRACTICES

In this chapter, self-care will include "testing the water" regarding activities you can do to be your own hypnotherapist. Pick a specific challenge you would like to face. You might want to improve on your relationships at work or with friends, a husband, or a wife. Assess your eating habits, exercise habits, sleep habits—whatever allows you to rejuvenate yourself and maintain daily balance. How is your attitude at home, after you've completed a long day of work? How is your attitude at work when you are overwhelmed and pushed to your limit? Begin making a list of all the traits you have that don't represent who you truly are. If you are a grump, put that trait on the list. Take time out and be honest with yourself, exploring the reasons why you choose to act this way (because it is a choice). After making your

Figure 5-1   My personal challenge list.

```
 1. _____
 2. _____
 3. _____
 4. _____
 5. _____
 6. _____
 7. _____
 8. _____
 9. _____
10. _____
11. _____
12. _____
13. _____
14. _____
15. _____
16. _____
17. _____
18. _____
19. _____
20. _____
```

Personal Challenge List (Fig. 5-1), choose a challenge to work on. You can always go back and work with more challenges on your list. For now, work on one challenge at a time until you are more comfortable with the process.

Relaxation Exercise

Description

Hypnosis works well because one of the steps in the process is to create a relaxed state of being. When we are in a relaxed state, we are able to receive suggestions that allow us to make needed changes. There are many types of relaxation exercises, but we will keep things simple. Progressive relaxation, visualization, and breathing exercises can be helpful in taking you to a place of peace. If you have another favorite relaxation technique, feel free to incorporate that into your experience also. We will practice relaxing ourselves and also being relaxed by a recording that we make ourselves.

Benefits

The exercises described here can help you master the art of relaxation *now*. After you practice them repeatedly, you can relax anytime and anyplace. You can relax at the drop of a hat, so to speak, which is very necessary when stressful situations arise at home and in the workplace. Relaxation helps you go within and find a place of calm. If you can access this place quickly, you can find solutions to many problems. Relaxation also helps with pain relief and insomnia. You can keep your immune system strong, boosted, and healthy because stress isn't depleting your adrenal glands. The benefits are endless.

Steps

Progressive muscle relaxation exercise

1. Make yourself comfortable and cozy, sitting or lying down.
2. Begin by tensing up all the muscles in your face, then relaxing them.
3. Tense the muscles in your neck and shoulders, then relax them.
4. Tense the muscles in your torso and abdomen, then relax them.
5. Tense the muscles in your thighs and buttocks, then relax them.
6. Tense the muscles in your upper legs, then relax them.
7. Tense the muscles in your calves, then relax them.
8. Tense the muscles in your ankles and feet, then relax them.
9. Tense your entire body, then relax.

(There are many variations to these relaxation exercises. You can do one extremity at a time, instead of both.)

Visualization exercise

1. Make yourself comfortable, sitting or lying down.
2. Let your mind take you to someplace peaceful and calming for you, such as a nice green pasture, a meadow, an enchanted forest, a mountain, or a beach.
3. Allow yourself to be relaxed there, feeling safe and at peace with your surroundings.
4. Continue to hold this feeling of peace, allowing it to fill up your body.

Counting Up and Deep Breathing exercise

1. Find a comfortable place for yourself, sitting or lying down.
2. Take in a nice deep breath through your nose.
3. As you take in that deep breath, hold it for 10 seconds (1, 1000, 2, 1000, etc.)
4. Exhale the breath through the mouth.
5. Repeat this process of breathing in and out five times.

6. Now begin counting from one, telling yourself you will be more and more relaxed.
7. Count to two, and tell yourself you will become more and more relaxed.
8. Count to three, four,...10 (with 10 being more relaxed than ever).

Practice any variation of these relaxation exercises to start. The more you practice them, the easier it will be to achieve relaxation. It can't be emphasized enough that these are things that can be done at a moment's notice, when you need calmness and clarity quickly.

Creating a Relaxation Script

If you have a recorder, you can record the relaxation script given below by simply reading it into the recorder. Feel free to be creative. There are no rules to this activity. You can play your favorite music in the background while you record this script. This makes the experience more personalized and allows your subconscious to really take note. Once you have recorded it, you can play it back to yourself and begin furthering your relaxation experience. Practice as many times as you can daily, in the morning and before you go to bed. If you don't have a recorder, you can make use of a volunteer in your home to read the relaxation script to you while you relax. You can also read the script to your partner in exchange, so you both can get the benefits of relaxation. When you are ready, practice writing your own script for relaxation. It can be so much fun to create scripts, share them with others, and watch a new dimension of your life unfold. The benefits of being able to stay calm and collected can be priceless. You are well on your way.

Relaxation script

Sit comfortably in a chair. Sit with your spine straight, feet flat on the floor, knees resting slightly apart. Your hands are resting comfortably in your lap or at your sides, with the palms comfortably facing up. Pick a place in your room to focus on for a minute. It can be a spot on the wall, a picture, or a light—whatever you choose. Put your attention on that place or object and become very aware of it. Begin breathing in through your nose and out through your mouth while focusing on the object. (Note: Place your hands on your stomach to make sure you are breathing correctly; your stomach should rise when you inhale and go down when you exhale.) Continue this breathing for six more cycles, breathing in through the nose and out through the mouth.

Now let your eyes close gently. Let your focus of attention move to your feet, which are flat on the floor. Curl your toes and tense your feet as tightly as you can. Take a breath in through your nose and hold that breath for 8 seconds. Now exhale the breath and release your feet, relaxing your toes, and allow the tension to melt away from your feet, sinking into the ground. Flex your feet and begin tightening the calves of your legs, with toes pointing toward you. Take a deep breath and hold it for 8 seconds while you experience the tension in the back of your legs. Exhale and allow the relaxation to flow down your legs as stress and tension leave your body.

Now begin to straighten your legs in front of you, lifting them slightly off the floor, locking your knees, and tightening your thigh muscles. Take a deep breath in through your nose, hold for 8 seconds, and exhale. Allow your legs to rest gently, letting the tension leave your body. Thank these parts of your body for the role they play in your physical functions. Allow gratitude to fill your thighs, your legs, and your feet. Feel a wave of relaxation go down your thighs, legs, and feet. Enjoy this feeling. Continue breathing in through the nose and out through the mouth, feeling more and more relaxed. Become aware of your arms and hands resting comfortably at your sides. Begin to extend your fingers in a nice stretch, flexing the palms, and hold for 8 seconds.

Now let your breath out. Extend your arms straight in front of you and ball your hands into a fist. Inhale your breath and hold for 8 seconds. Now exhale through the mouth and relax. Become aware of your arms. Your attention is now going to the forearms and the upper arms. Inhale and hold your breath for 8 seconds. Now exhale the breath and relax, allowing your arms and hands to drop. Your hands are heavy, palms are facing upward, and you feel like a rag doll just lying there and being very relaxed. Continue breathing in through your nose and out through your mouth. Give your attention to your shoulders. Lift your shoulders up to meet your ears. Lift your shoulders up to meet your ears and keep them there as you begin to inhale, and hold your breath for 8 seconds. When you release the breath, begin to let your shoulders drop. Your awareness is now being shifted to your back. Picture a beautiful balloon attached to the front of your chest. The balloon begins to fly away, and as it flies away it lifts your chest toward the sky. Let your back arch and lift toward the sky. As your spine arches, inhale for 8 seconds. Relax the spine as you exhale and release the breath. Feel a deep sense of relaxation in your spine, as it rests in your chair. Place your awareness on your torso. Tighten your stomach and chest, drawing in your chest muscles and sucking in your stomach muscles at the same time. Take a deep breath in and hold that breath for 8 seconds. Relax your chest muscles and then your stomach muscles, feeling an even greater calmness come over your body.

Feel the gratitude you have for the parts of your body you have just relaxed and thank them for their service to you. Focus now on your neck; begin a neck roll, gently going clockwise and then counterclockwise. Do this one more time and feel the relaxation. Tighten your neck muscles, inhale, and hold your breath for 8 seconds. Now release the tension in your neck, exhale the breath, and do another gentle neck roll for deeper relaxation. Place your attention on your face now. Push your tongue against the roof of your mouth, make your jaws tighten, and hold your teeth together. Inhale and hold your breath for 8 seconds, then exhale into deep peace. Now take a deep breath in and open your mouth as if you are yawning. Leave your mouth open for 8 seconds; feel your cheeks and lips stretching. Now exhale, allowing your face and chin to relax, and let the feeling of deeper relaxation nurture you. You are feeling so deeply relaxed now. Every inhalation nourishes your body. Every exhalation cleanses your body. Allow yourself to bask in the peace, the clarity, the serenity, and the calmness you feel right now. There is no need to do anything at this point, other than to relax and just be aware of the moment.

Negativity Observation Exercise

To be able to change our habits or improve our behaviors, we must face what our limitations are and turn those limitations into victories. Negativity limits us from being the very best that we can be, and is a challenge we are often faced with on a daily basis at home or at work. It is very difficult to describe negativity. When we experience an adverse occurrence or interaction, our perception of it coupled with our response to it can give rise to negativity. We definitely know that it doesn't feel good to the body, the mind, or spirit; however, negativity is a choice. We can choose to be positive or negative in any challenging situation that arises. Another interesting point about negativity is that it is contagious. It can spread like a bad rash. People may approach us in ways that we feel are wrong, because of our belief systems, cultural backgrounds, status, etc. We then take that event and process it. "Hey, they don't need to treat me this way!" The ball begins to roll from there. You can either score a basket or go out of bounds. There is definitely a process involved in dealing with negativity. It is like stop, drop, and roll. Stop, think, and respond with compassion (not react). I am not one for superstitions, but if you happen to get out of bed on the "wrong" side, you might want to consciously get back in bed and complete the process again. Get out on the side you believe is the "right" one and go on to create the joyous day you were meant to have, and share that joy with others.

You may work in an environment that could be considered toxic or highly negative. It may be a place where much gossiping occurs, and people are trying to climb the career ladder. In striving for success, they may feel it is necessary to make others look bad, to make themselves look good. Some toxic environments have management personnel who are unapproachable and very demeaning to the staff. The staff or employees may have personal problems that they take out on their coworkers because they don't know how to cope with the situations. To make the choice to be different in this type of environment requires a great deal of self-awareness and self-care of your mental state. Positivity is when we see the bright side of things, are more apt to work toward solutions, and are encouraging and supportive of others. Do you believe achieving positivity is easier said than done? If you answer "yes," then you might be feeling helpless and doubtful that you or others can change. Baby steps are all that is needed right now. All we really need is the intent to change. It is not in our nature to want to be negative; however, certain situations can shift us toward negativity if we don't take time to recognize and assess our own personal feelings right away. Negativity is expressed in attitudes, behaviors, words, and expressions that cause us to have adverse reactions to situations, ourselves, or other people.

For the purpose of our exercises, we are going to be looking at ourselves from the outside. We are going to determine how we bring negativity to others. We immediately recognize when we have been wronged, misjudged, and treated unfairly. Do we recognize or even acknowledge when we bring a negative energy into the settings and interactions we are involved in? This is definitely a learning experience, and you should be very gentle with yourself. It is not what happens to us, it is how we respond to what happens that creates the greatest impact in our lives.

Rubber-band exercise

Description

I learned about the rubber-band exercise at a seminar conducted by a colleague. Find a rubber band that fits around your wrist like a bracelet, making sure it is not too lose or too tight (you should be able to fit a pinky finger between your wrist and the rubber band). From the time you wake up in the morning to the time you go to bed, you are going to be conscious of your thoughts, actions toward others, and interactions with others. Each time you think something that is mean, sarcastic, or degrading about another person, give that rubber band a snap. Each time you think something that is mean, sarcastic, or degrading about yourself, give that rubber band a little pop. Any time you feel the urge to vent about someone who is not being helpful in solving a problem, give the rubber band a pop. Each time you think you are right, just because you think so, you will be closed off to other options or solutions to the issue. Give the rubber band a snap.

We have an inner mechanism that allows us to know deep inside when we are out of harmony with others. This mechanism is called a conscience. The rubber-band exercise is not a punishment for you by any means, to cause your wrist to be blistered by the end of the day. This is a discrete action that you can do anywhere that allows you to become more aware of your own personal seeds of negativity that you might be sowing in different places you frequent. (If snapping doesn't resonate with you, you can put a dime in a jar each time you are negative. If you happen to fill that jar up, bless the money and give the proceeds to charity. People will not be benefitting from your negativity, but rather from your learning and awareness.) You will know whether you are reaching for that rubber band a lot or a little, by the end of the day. Keep a journal of your experience and record each time you became aware that you were acting in negative ways toward yourself and others.

Benefits

The benefit to this exercise is self-awareness. We begin to take responsibility for the roles we play at work and at home, and how we fit into the solutions. If we are aware of how we allow negativity to creep into situations, we are that much more empowered to stop it right then and there.

Steps

1. Find or purchase a rubber band. (I like to purchase colored rubber bands and pick a color according to my needs on a particular day, as a little bonus color therapy.)
2. Do not get a rubber band that cuts off the circulation in your wrist. We want you to keep your wrist for future use.
3. Snap the rubber band throughout the day when you experience opportunities to be negative.

   - Snap your rubber band when you think of things that are negative and don't serve you (i.e., things that are destructive and don't work to build you or others up as human beings).
   - Snap your rubber band when you act on the thoughts you have to be negative or do negative things to others.
   - Snap your rubber band if you say things about yourself or others that are harmful or defaming.
   - Snap your rubber band if you feel like you are smarter, better, brighter, prettier, or more efficient than others.
   - You get the point.

4. At the end of the day, do a snap tally. Don't be discouraged if your snap tally goes through the roof (like in the hundreds). What we are going for now is to achieve consciousness and self-awareness of how we contribute to the negativity in our environment.
5. You can record each experience you have or the experiences that stand out for you. You can summarize the experiences you felt and express what you learned from them. Feel free to express yourself in any way you choose.
6. Thank your wrists for their participation in your self-awareness project. Most importantly, thank yourself for being open to growth and change.

Forgive yourself for the negativity you have carried within yourself and shared with others.

7. Visualize yourself being different and able to demonstrate positivity when you are faced with situations that are difficult. Set your intention to do something different.

Positive Suggestions Exercise

What your mind focuses on will come to pass, whether it be positive or negative. In the previous exercise, we became aware of negativity and its impact. Positivity is just as contagious as negativity. If we are used to being negative about situations, achieving positivity will require practice, but it can be done if we work at it. Positivity can and should be seen as a natural part of living and communicating with others. Positivity comes in many different forms. You can be thankful for what you have. You can praise others for what they are doing right. You can look at your accomplishments and acknowledge yourself as a creator. You can practice communicating with others in compassionate ways that build relationships instead of tearing them down.

Description

There are a few exercises we can do to develop positivity. First, we will make a gratitude list. This list will include all the things you are grateful for in this world. You can go through all the people you know and begin to pick out reasons why you are grateful for them. Think of all the experiences you are currently facing, and write down what you are grateful for in those circumstances. Think about yourself and your family, spouse, kids, parents, siblings, job, patients, and coworkers; think about people you admire, or good things that are happening in the world. Go for it! This exercise can keep you busy for a lifetime.

Benefits

Gratitude is a big component of self-change. If you can look at your situation and see the good in it, you will become much more creative in dealing with challenges and conflict. Gratitude puts you in the channel to attract the things you desire, because you are grateful for what you have. You will also attract more people into your life who have similar goals and desires. This is not to say that you will never interact with a difficult person ever again, just because you are grateful. It means that you will be able to keep your perspective and possibly be the light in that person's life that causes change. Your days may not be easier, but they will be more enjoyable, and you won't be fazed by the challenges that come. You will be a creator, a beacon of positive light.

If we are able to keep a positive outlook, we can create success in our lives. Our environments will be better, and our relationships and interactions with others will be improved. Our body will feel better because we are not harboring emotions that lead to illness, mental duress, and disease.

Steps

Take out your journal or a sheet of paper and make a list of all the things and people you are grateful for. Keep going until you feel you have tapped yourself out. Take note of how you feel after making your list. Reflect on it often, especially when you feel the world is an awful place to be. Add to this list daily as things come to you that you may not have included in the first round.

Different Forms of Suggestion

Suggestions are an important factor in hypnosis. We receive suggestions every single day from ourselves and from the people we interact with daily. We have received suggestions from our parents, teachers, friends, coworkers, and family every single day of our lives. Some of those suggestions have been productive, while others have not. Nevertheless, those suggestions have contributed to who we are.

According to Caprio and Berger (1998), there are many ways in which we receive suggestions. We can receive suggestions directly. Direct suggestions are given in a commanding manner and are straight to the point. An example would be, "Answer my call light, now!" We also receive suggestions indirectly. Indirect suggestions are mainly nonverbal, and may even be sounds or visual cues that we might find ourselves responding to without being aware we are doing so. For example, when you look down on the ground because you have dropped something, other people often begin to look down at the ground also. Suggestions by inference are subtle and nonverbal, and may involve motion. For example, you ask your patient if he or she understands what you're saying, and they nod their head. This nodding indicates understanding. Another form of receiving suggestions is emotional appeal. For example, if you wish to clear a crowded room, you can simply yell, "Fire!" The tone of your voice and the yelling will cause a panic among people in the room. Suggestions by social dictates are those we receive from trends, fashions, slang, politics, etc. (for example, not too long ago, bell-bottoms were fashionable and everyone was wearing them). Negative cliché suggestions are constantly instilled in our minds; we come to believe them and expect nothing less than what has been stated. Examples of this would include "No pain, no gain," "Life is short and then you die," and "You need money to get ahead in life." There are negative suggestions that create physical manifestations, such as, "My husband is a pain in the neck," or "That patient is driving me crazy!" Eventually you get a little neck pain here and there, you're seeing a chiropractor every other week, and you're wondering what is wrong with your body.

There is also a category of positive suggestions, which suggest that something will take place no matter what. The phrase "I will..." generally is not used in hypnotherapy because it leaves a goal to be met in the future. It doesn't help the mind see it as being completed. Telling yourself "I will graduate from nursing school" is like saying "I will graduate from nursing school someday in the future." Telling yourself "I am a graduate of nursing school" gets your brain thinking that it needs to create this for you because it has already been done. Get the picture?

Suggestion Exercise

Creating suggestions that are beneficial to your well-being may require some observance and practice on your part. Be mindful of what your thoughts and words are toward yourself and the goals you desire to accomplish in life. Take the opportunity to stop yourself when you are making negative suggestions, and rephrase anything that comes to your awareness.

Description

Go back to the personal challenge list you created earlier. Think of ways you can rephrase those traits you listed, to make them positive and self-affirming. You have the power to transform yourself into the person you desire, so you are going to take each trait and change it to something your subconscious mind will create for you. Take, for example, "I am a grump!" This is not how you wish to be or how you wish to relate to others. You can rephrase this to "I am friendly, I am cordial, I am a joy to be around!" When you create the suggestions you wish to see manifested in your life, you must be positive, specific, and very detailed. Keep your suggestions in the present tense, as if they are occurring right now. Use creative and exciting words that will stand out in your mind, but be realistic. "I am dull and unattractive" can be changed to "I am exuberant and flattering to myself and others." If you have 25 cents in your bank account, don't give yourself a suggestion that you will be a millionaire tomorrow. Your brain would laugh you off the face of the earth. Your mind can create that situation for you over time, however, and the proper suggestion would be "I increase increase in wealth daily." Complete the list of personal traits and transform those traits into what you truly desire to be like. Once you have completed that list, explore situations, relationships, and circumstances in your life you would also like to change.

Benefits

This exercise helps you to get deep down to you who are and what you want to be, and to realize the power you have to change yourself. You will focus less on what others are doing to you, because you will develop an awareness of what you are already doing to yourself. This is the exercise that tears up your front yard. However, after you have raked the yard thoroughly and put a little grass seed down (positive suggestions), you will have green grass in no time! Your yard at home and your yard at work will be greener, fuller, and thicker because you are tending to them in a very special way. It might seem scary at first to read what's on your list. You may feel like you're somewhat of a mess or there is nothing good about yourself at all. This is what needs to come out, because it is definitely impacting your relationships, profession, and self-image. The best benefit of this exercise is that you will realize you have nothing to be ashamed of and nothing to hide or hide from.

Self-Hypnosis Script Exercise

Now we get to put all the different things we have learned and practiced into play. Most importantly, we know how to relax. We can visualize, breathe, and relax with muscle progression. We are aware of the negative and positive things we think and say, and how they impact the brain. We are aware of how suggestions are received in positive and negative ways, and how to create suggestions for our own image. These are all the important components to making our own hypnosis script.

Description

Steps

A self-hypnosis script consists of four parts: the relaxation phase, the suggestive phase, the visualization phase, and finally the counting-down and waking-up phase. Now you will create your own script based on what you wish to immediately accomplish in life. For example, you can pick weight reduction as the issue for your hypnosis script. Pick the type of relaxation that is most appealing for you. Take the positive suggestions you have created based on the weight issue, or create positive suggestions that deal with management. Create a space in your script in which you allow yourself to visualize the "you" that you desire to see. Finally, you will do a reversal of the relaxation exercise and wake yourself up (an example of this will be given in the script.) The script does not have to be long. It can be direct and to the point.

Benefits

The main benefit of this exercise is self-empowerment. You are taking control of your life, career, and issues that you might not have had the courage to deal with before. Things that may have interfered with how you related to others and felt about yourself or your career can be expressed and reveal things to you for your learning experience.

My Weight Reduction Script

*RELAXATION*_____*(insert your relaxation exercise of choice)*
*SUGGESTION*_____*(insert your suggestions of choice)*

Sample Suggestions:

- I am the right weight for my body.
- I am strong, healthy, and slender.
- My body readily burns the fat I have stored.
- I enjoy the foods that are good for me.
- I enjoy green, leafy vegetables.
- I take in exactly what my body needs.
- My body has no need for extra fat.
- I enjoy fruits and vegetables daily.
- I enjoy daily exercise.
- I enjoy drinking water to cleanse my system.
- The craving for sweets has diminished.
- The urge for sweets lessens daily.
- Foods that harm my body are undesirable to me.

Visualization

Here is an example of a visualization you can include in your script. Personalize your visualization for the topic you have chosen.

Imagine yourself at the mall. You reward yourself for your weight reduction with an outfit to wear for an event. You feel so good about the changes you are making for yourself and your body; you thoroughly are enjoying this event. You see the clothes on the racks, you see clothes on the clearance racks, and you see clothes folded on the display that are so appealing to you and your style. You find clothes your size in all these places and you smile with gratitude. You no longer dread the dressing room or asking for help in picking out something to wear. You find an attendant and ask her for help. She smiles at you and says she has an outfit in mind that will be so flattering for you. You experience excitement and anticipation as she goes to find you an outfit. She returns to you with three sizes. One size bigger than what you wear, one size is what you think you might be, and one size is smaller than what you might currently wear. You give her back the bigger size and decide that you will try on the other two. You realize that you are on a path to weight reduction, and there are no disappointments because you are always doing what is best for you. You try on the size that you feel is right for you, because it looks like it will fit. Wow! You look great, but there is some space in the dress. You would have to take it in if you purchased it. You take it off and realize that the next option is the smaller dress. You try that dress on. It is now the perfect size for you. You stand in front of the mirror. You admire your body, you love your body, and you love yourself, even when you are standing in front of the dressing room mirror. With each outfit you try on, you acknowledge that it is a smaller size than what you used to wear in the past. You feel good about your shopping, because you have taken care of your body in many amazing ways. Your dedication to yourself has made this moment possible and enjoyable for you.

Wake-Up Exercise

The wake-up exercise basically recaps everything you have experienced in working on your script. You are summarizing and counting up to get your body more aware and awake from the self-hypnosis process. Then your mind can process all the work you have done, while you go on with your day. If you are doing this at night, you can tell yourself that you will simply fall asleep as the work is being done.

You have experienced a great deal of progress. You are determined to reach your goals through your dedication. The road ahead is very possible and easy. Weight reduction is easy, and you prove it every day with every pound you throw away and with every inch that comes off your waste and hips. You are more excited about yourself and your life, and are able to accomplish many more things because of the way you have improved in your eating and exercise habits. Now it is time to begin bringing your body back to awareness. Begin counting from 10 down to 1. As you count, feel the sensation coming back to your hands and feet. Your body is beginning to feel that it is time to get up now, as you gradually are becoming more alert and aware. You could open your eyes anytime you want, but you are awakening slowly, to be gentle to your body. You have so much gratitude for the success of your process and what your mind can accomplish. You are now at one; now open your eyes!

Sample scripts are illustrated in the following figures:

Energy and vitality (Fig. 5-2)

Compassion (Fig. 5-3)

Releasing fear (Fig. 5-4)

Self-care (Fig. 5-5)

These scripts are meant to be used in conjunction with the relaxation techniques you have learned. Feel free to write your own script. Just think about what you want to accomplish and talk to your mind!

Figure 5-2   Energy and vitality script.

Fatigue is a sign that we are out of balance somewhere in our lives. If we are tired and exhausted, we might not have gotten the right amount of rest, eaten the right foods, or done other things that keep us feeling alive and vibrant. Let's back track and look at ourselves. Let's look at our day to day actions and see if we see a place where we might be losing energy. Do you see it? Do you feel the leak that is draining you of precious energy or life force? If it is your job, explore what must be done to capture your energy. If it is your family, explore what you must do to reclaim the energy. Do you need to be more honest, more organized, more assertive? What things will help you to regain the energy that you are losing? When you are ready, begin to seal those leaks that you have. Whatever the cause of the leak, know that you have the power to seal the leaks and create a life full of vibrancy, health, and energy for yourself. You have the energy and vitality you need to meet the daily activities in your life. You have the energy and vitality to have fun. You have the energy and vitality to do your work. You have mastered the balance between work and home, because you take care of yourself. From this point on, you have the ability to notice the leaks before you lose your life force energy. All you need to do is go within, anytime and any-where. All you have to do is take a deep breath and know that you are complete. Feel the energy and life force return to you. It's that simple, because you have made it that simple. You are full of energy and vitality and it's awesome!

Self-Hypnosis Tape Activity (Part 2)

Description

Record the script so that you can continue to listen to it any time you want to. Over time, you can create scripts for other areas you desire to work on and record them as well. This way you can hear them over and over again, and they become instilled in your subconscious mind.

Steps

Record the script you have written in your own voice and play it during your break time, in the morning, or at night before you go to bed.

Benefits

Your subconscious mind will set out to make the things you are working toward happening, allowing you to achieve success in reaching your goals.

Figure 5-3   Compassion.

People make their own choices and live their lives their own ways. Sometimes their actions impact us in ways that seem adverse and sometimes annoying. How do we care for people who might be irresponsible or seem like they don't care about themselves or others around them? Think back in your mind and go back as far as you need to in time. Has there ever been a time in your life when you have made poor choices? Did those choices impact others in unfortunate ways? What was that like? How did you feel? Did you forget about it and pretend like it never happened? Were you embarrassed that you ever behaved in that way? Those were a lot of questions. Take your time and think about them carefully. We recognize many things in others, because we are capable of doing them ourselves. Because we have the same potential, we can still help others to be responsible for their actions, but we can do it in a way that plants a seed. Compassion is a seed that helps us to know that know of us are perfect, but we can grow out of patterns that don't serve us and change. See yourself planting seeds in the lives of others. The seeds of compassion grow and blossom. There is no judgment, no anger, and no resentment for what others do. You are not responsible for it. You are responsible for your truth, honesty, and concern that you plant into lives by being who you are. That feels so much better than hoarding negative energy around concerning people that you want to change to be what you want them to be. It is much easier to plant the seeds and walk away. You don't overwater the plant or nurture it to death. You simply walk away and let it grow. When you turn around, the possibilities are endless. Regardless of the outcomes you have compassion and care for people unconditionally and with love.

Figure 5-4   Releasing fear.

Fear is false evidence appearing real. We know this. That is why we are here and ready to face our fears. A bible scripture says that "The Lord has not given us the spirit of fear, but of power, of love, and of a sound mind." What is fear? Fear is a feeling of dread for something we cannot see or control. What can we do to help rid ourselves of fear? We can look at reality. The emotions of worry, doubt, anger, sadness, trying too hard are things that aren't necessary for us to hold on to...ever! We release these feelings that plague our relationships at home and at work. We are enthusiastic about the future, because fear is

(continued)

Figure 5-4   *(continued)*

someplace far away. Negative emotions are a part of the past, because we know the source is fear. We know how to send fear on its way. Simply take a breath and invision yourself shoeing fear out with a pitchfork, because it has no place in your life. Fear does more harm and never does good, because it keeps you from doing what you need to remedy your situation. You have a creative brain that can solve any problem. Fear only stands in the way. You have a heart that can love others and build relationships. Fear only stands in the way. You have dreams that you want to accomplish. So guess who has to go. You are right! Fear get's the boot. You are successful. You can stay successful as long as fear is recognized for what it is. A nuisance. Love begins to find its way into the situation. Love fills in the dark shadows that fear once lurked in. Love illuminates your thoughts, your words, and your actions. Love has the power to stay. You keep yourself centered at all times. You are strong and recognize when an opportunity arises for fear to creep in. You recognize that you might have handled things differently in the past, but there is no guilt. There is no reason to repeat a past that didn't work either. You have a new pathway that serves you well. You choose the way of love over fear, every single time!

Figure 5-5   Self-care.

Once upon a time you might have felt it important to spend every minute of your day caring for others. You might have thought that it was your calling to be all things to everyone, every minute, and every where, every day. You may have been raised to be that service to mankind is worthy, but service to yourself is selfish. Let's clear something up now. Service to mankind is very worthy. We are here to help one another. The truth is that we can't be here, if we care less for ourselves. You started to notice the struggles that you were feeling when you couldn't meet the demands of everyone at all times. You no longer cared to be tired and resentful, because you had given so much of yourself. You found yourself saying things that you didn't mean, and taking on more responsibilities than you needed to for the last time. You have a life worth living. Your life honors self-care. There is a balance that you are entitled to in your life. There is a law of giving and receiving that gives you permission to take full part in self-care. Guilt free, because you deserve it! Take a deep breath and know that it is good that you feel that struggle. That struggle is an indicator that helped you to change your thinking and actions. Your body, mind, and spirit are sending you a constant message. This message is that it is okay to release the pressure of being the perfect caregiver. The truth is that we all do the best we can, but we don't have to be perfect. It is impossible. There is a beauty in being human. Because we are human, we have physical limitations that require us to take special care of ourselves too. That is why being a perfect caregiver, means being a perfect caregiver to ourselves first. You are a perfect caregiver, because you take care of yourself every single day in so many beautiful ways. Your eating habits reflect your self-care, because the fruits and vegetables you give your body are exactly what it needs. Your body takes a rest when it needs to and you have learned to listen to the messages your body sends you. You think thoughts of success, joy, and happiness about your life and you have a spirit of gratefulness for everything you do and experience. You take time to experience nature, you exercise often, and you nurture your spiritual man through meditation and prayer. It is easy for you to give to others, because you give so much to yourself. It is easy for you to spread joy to everyone, because you have a relationship with yourself that helps your joy to grow. Congratulations for being an example, for living a life of self-care, and being strong enough to learn from your past. Self-care is the most important daily routine you have. The world will see you and care for themselves too!

EXPERIENCING HYPNOTHERAPY AS A CLIENT

Selecting a Hypnotist/Hypnotherapist

Hypnosis schools do not come under state or federal regulations, so picking a hypnotherapist may require a little work on your part. There are hypnotists out there who advertise doctorates that are null and void because the programs were not accredited. Or they may have attained their credentials that is too short for a legitimate doctoral program. When selecting a hypnotherapist, consider whether he is licensed or nonlicensed. Some hypnotherapists are licensed and come from a background of psychology, nursing, medicine, social work, counseling, chiropractic, naturopathy, homeopathy, or some other professional category. Some say that therapists or hypnotists may have received training from a program but are not members of a licensed profession. This doesn't mean that they are not good hypnotists, but experience levels will vary with the background of the practitioner. Ask for references and information about their education and number of years in practice. A free consultation is always a plus because it gives you the opportunity to meet the therapist and get a feeling of his or her "vibes." Reputable Web sites list resources and training for hypnotists and can make recommendations for therapists in a geographical area. Holistic magazines and Web sites are also good sources for finding a hypnotherapist who would be interested in working with you.

Pricing for Sessions

Hypnotherapy sessions generally range from $50 to $250 (or more) per hour, depending on the practitioner's expertise and reputation, and the cost of living in a particular area.

Duration of Sessions

Sessions will generally last about 1 to 1.5 hours. Generally, the therapist will perform an intake interview before the session to inquire about the client's health history, including traumas, surgeries, medications, and mental illness. Certain medications and certain forms of mental illness must be taken into consideration when a person undergoes hypnotherapy. If a person has had brain trauma or a severe mental illness, I refer them to a psychologist or a psychiatrist. The intake interview is sometimes conducted over the phone. I like to do the intake about 2 to 5 days before the first session, so that I can review the client's history and allow my intuition to go to work on deciding what will be the best interventions for that person.

What to Expect From a Session

What you can expect from a session can vary. Some people expect "fireworks and bells" to go off, but that hardly ever happens. Nevertheless, the effects of hypnosis are still taking place. You may not really feel like you have been hypnotized until later, when you begin to notice the changes that you have been seeking. At the time I was completing my training, I hypnotized a friend who was interested in weight management. I suggested to her that she would love skim milk, as opposed to the whole milk she had been guzzling down for so long. She went to the store and saw the skim milk. She decided "not today," and reached for the whole milk. The next day, when she prepared some cereal for her children, she noticed that she had actually purchased the skim milk! She didn't feel like she had been hypnotized, because the process was so subtle. However, the subconscious mind was there and took good notes about what took place. All I can say is, keep an open mind. You can expect relaxation. You will do quite a bit of talking to the hypnotherapist. Problem solving takes place from your own perspective, as you look at your issues and challenges. You will also experience a lot of visualization and affirmation that will give your mind a different and more expansive perspective.

FURTHER STUDIES IN HYPNOSIS

Hypnotherapy Training

I attended the Missouri Institute of Hypnotherapy and my instructor was Linda Gentry, a registered nurse who also has a degree in psychology. My experience with Linda was very meaningful and entertaining because she also happens to be a stage hypnotist. Her stories opened me up to many career possibilities if nursing didn't work out! The prices for hypnotherapy programs range from hundreds to thousands of dollars. My program was in a seminar setting that offered continuing-education units. We were asked to read many books, complete homework assignments, and perform clinical exercises on our classmates, family, and friends. Linda seemed to eat, drink, and breathe hypnotherapy every single day. This made the difference in my choosing her training. This should also be a consideration for you, should you decide to pursue training in hypnotherapy.

Hypnotherapy Associations

Hypnotherapy associations are good sources for finding training programs, resources, and referrals to hypnotherapists. They can help you find what the standards are for hypnotherapists, check credentials, and explore the qualifications to make sure you are getting the best experience you possibly can. Below are listed some of these associations and their Web sites:

International Alliance of Professional Hypnotists: www.hypnosisalliance.com

International Association of Counselors and Therapists: www.iact.org

National Guild of Hypnotists: www.ngh.net

Missouri Institute of Hypnotherapy: www.hypnosismo.com

American Hypnosis Association: www.hypnosis.edu

American International Association of Hypnosis: www.choosehypnosis.com

International Hypnosis Association: www.hypnosiscredentials.com

REFERENCES

Ansari, M. (1991). *Modern hypnosis: Theory and practice*. Washington, DC: Mass-Press.

Caprio, F., & Berger, J. R. (1998). *Healing yourself with self-hypnosis*. Paramus, NJ: Prentice Hall Press.

SUGGESTED READING LIST

Fallon, S. (2001). *Nourishing traditions*. Washington, DC: New Trends Publishing.

Libster, M. (2002). *Delmar's integrative herb guide for nurses*. Albany, NY: Delmar Publishing Company.

CHAPTER 6

Introduction to the Chakra System

RACHEL Y. HILL

"There is a deep wisdom within our very flesh, if we can only come to our senses and feel it."
—ELIZABETH A. BEHNKE

I have done some quirky things to keep myself motivated to get a job done. Writing this book was fun, but sometimes it was a challenge to keep my thoughts flowing in ways they should. And although writing it was truly a labor of love, I decided I needed a ritual to make this experience less about the labor and more about the love. I didn't know how I would do this, but I set the intention to find a ritual for my book-writing experience. Shortly after setting my intention, I went to my local office supply store for a few items. I should tell you that for me, being in an office supply store is similar to the experience of a child being locked in a room with a 5-pound bag of candy for 15 minutes. You'd probably be surprised at how much candy a child can consume in 15 minutes. You'd be even more surprised at how many office supplies, pens, and gadgets I can buy in 15 minutes. This time I was searching for printer paper. I was in the paper section and just happened to come upon the most magnificent colored paper I had ever seen. The paper stood out like a neon light, and the realization hit me suddenly: This is your ritual! The colored paper would be my fun reward for writing, and the ritual I would use to complete my book.

The colors were exciting and fun for me. Even if I sat down feeling tired, I would finish up my writing feeling energized and excited about what I would be sharing with you. The colors were from the rainbow. These colors are also the colors of the chakra, with each color standing for a particular theme of our human existence. Each time I sat down to write, I would choose a different color I was drawn to at that time. The colors kept things fun and exciting for me throughout the entire writing process. Interestingly enough, the ritual began to take on a different meaning for me—more than simple excitement and fun. The more I thought about the different colors I was choosing for my purposes, I realized that I was drawing the colors in that I needed for my own personal balance and harmony. I also found myself using colored ink pens and taking notice of which color I chose. My quirky ritual turned out to be a wonderful exercise in self-observation. I would close my eyes and pick a colored ink pen out of my bag; then I would close my eyes and ask myself, What color of paper should I write on today? The color would appear in my mind's eye, and that would begin my ritual. The self-observation would come in when I would reflect on the meanings of the colors I chose, determine what chakra I needed to give attention to in my life, and begin my writing experience aware of what I needed to give myself as I shared with you. Pretty neat, isn't it?

INTRODUCTION TO THE CHAKRA SYSTEM

The chakra system is an ancient system that dates back to more than 5000 years ago. As with other ancient healing forms, the chakra system was at risk of being forgotten. This tradition was carried on through generations by many written works and also by word of mouth; however, with the major transitions of civilization and war, much of that information was either destroyed or lost. We are very fortunate to have the information on the chakra system we have today and the various individuals who spend a great deal of time studying that system. We can consider ourselves very blessed to have what we have been able to glean from the ancient writings and oral tradition. As deeper insights from this information reemerge, it is very easy to learn something new and exciting about ourselves each and every day. Through ancient writings and oral tradition, we have been able to learn a great deal about our existence within, and how it relates to the world outside ourselves. According to Anodea Judith (1987), the connection between the chakra system and the science of yoga can be traced through various ancient writings. The Vedas (Veda is Sanskrit for "knowledge") comprise one of the oldest collections of texts in India. In these writings, reference is made to the chakras. The writings are said to have stemmed from the Aryans, an Indo-European tribe that traveled through India in the second millennium BCE. Chakra means sacred wheel or discs (Judith, 1987), and stems from the wheels of the invading Aryans' chariots.

Concept of the Chakra System

Every living being in this world is full of energy or the life force. That means anything that breathes, walks, crawls, snores, and grows is full of this life energy. An energy field is emitted from every living being that is very subtle. This energy is considered putative, because it is difficult to measure. Some people can see this energy and the colors that are dominant within the field at a particular time. Some can feel the energy with their hands. Some can pick up impressions, just by knowing within themselves that this energy exists. The aura has often been visualized in artwork as a glow or halo, such as those seen on depictions of Jesus, saints, angels, and other enlightened beings who once walked the earth. The aura is emitted from the body, but comes from the chakras spinning collectively.

According to Bruyere (1994), "Our auric or electromagnetic field is generated by the spinning of the chakras." The artists who painted those beautiful pictures either saw the auras themselves or had an understanding from what others shared with them about what they were able to see, and painted the pictures in faith that such a glow exists. For those of us who are unable to see auras, Kirlian photography can be used to capture the auras of individuals. This is how we know that this biofield is something that is very real. "Kirlian photography is a new field of research for Western medical science; however, numerous practitioners in eastern Europe use this diagnostic technique (which they term bioelectrography). Physical and emotional health and disease can be identified in plants, animals, and humans using this method" (Koopsen & Young, 2009).

Many of us might feel limited in our understanding because we do not think we are sensitive to energy at all. However, there are many ways in which we are sensing energy all the time; we are just not aware that we are actually doing it. Have you ever been sleeping and felt the need to wake up and open your eyes, only to find someone standing over you? You sensed a presence or energy and were moved to awaken. When someone walks into a room, you look up and see him or her, feel his or her presence, and determine whether he or she is someone you are drawn to or not. Rub your hands together really fast, back and forth for 5 seconds. Stop and hold your hands about an inch apart. Note what you feel. Do you feel a vibration? Do you feel a pulling? Do you feel anything at all? Separate your hands a little further, taking note. Continue to separate your hands further until you are unable to feel anything at all. Know that if you did feel something, it was merely your body's own energy field.

Why do we need to talk about auras during our discussion on chakras? The aura must be discussed in conjunction with chakras because the aura is created by the chakras as a collective whole. According to Bruyere (1994), "The seven major chakras are located along a central axis parallel to the spinal column of the physical body." These seven chakras or energy centers align to form a vertical column called the sushuna. The energy centers can be described as spinning vortexes of light that join together to form the electromagnetic field of the body (the aura). The aura is often described as a golden, white, or colorful glow around an individual. The chakras are represented by specific beautiful colors. Those who are able to see the auras of others usually are seeing the colors of the chakras that are the most dominant within the individual's energy field at that time. This is where Kirlian photography is often used. The aura varies in its size, shape, and color. It can be a healthy color based on the chakra's function within the body, or it can present an unhealthy picture. In other words, the aura can be no better than the chakras' ability to function. The adequate functioning of the chakras determines the quality of the aura. If the aura looks unhealthy, it is likely that something is going on with the chakras, and thus with the body as well.

Figure 6-1   Chakra image.

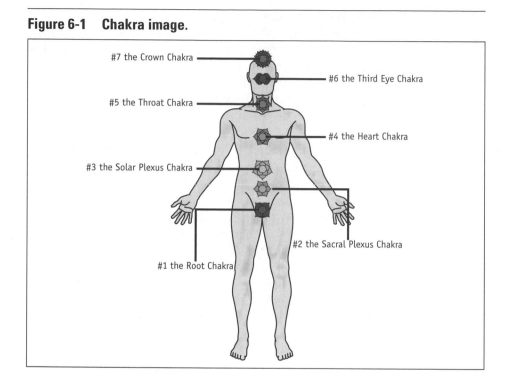

Figure 6-1 illustrates the chakras and their placement on the physical body. The beauty of understanding the chakras is that we can detect disharmony within our mental, spiritual, and physical states. When the chakras are out of balance, we can detect things that are going on with our physical bodies, our thoughts, and our experiences. With adequate understanding of each chakra and function, we can correct these imbalances by changing our thoughts, lifestyle, and environments. Without this knowledge of the chakras, we may go on living day to day in disharmony, and illnesses are likely to result from these imbalances. Each chakra is linked to a body system and an endocrine gland, so disharmony that impacts the chakra will soon appear to impact the body.

A person could spend a lifetime studying the chakras. Feel free to delve deeper into this system, but the basics to get you started will definitely go a long way. For the chakra system to remain harmonious, it must be balanced. There are many ways in which the chakras can be balanced. The energy therapies we have discussed all have balancing effects on the chakra system. Reiki impacts the chakras because the Reiki practitioner works in the fields where the chakras rest. Normal chakra function is indicated by a clockwise spin of the chakra. Why do we need to keep the chakras balanced and spinning clockwise? When they aren't spinning in a clockwise fashion, it means they are dysfunctional. They can be either too open or too closed, as indicated by the wheels spinning too fast (excessive) or too slowly (deficient). When these dysfunctions occur, disease and emotional imbalance are sure to be evident.

According to Bruyere (1994), the chakras cannot be either opened or closed. Many people try to describe the chakras as being open or closed; however, what they actually are trying to describe is the energy level of each chakra. The energy is either a lot more or less than what is within balance for each individual. Imagine a flat tire. It is difficult to drive with such a tire because it doesn't have enough air to create the pressure to keep the tire inflated so that it can roll. With too much air in the tire, however, other problems can occur that affect the balance of the vehicle (your body). The tire gauge is the means by which you check your tires so that you can make the proper adjustments and let more air in or more air out.

As mentioned previously, we know that some people have the ability to see the chakras. There are other ways in which we can detect the presence of the chakras in our bodies. Some people are able to feel the chakras with the palms of their hands, which enables them to detect the motion in which the chakra is spinning. Some people are able to know this intuitively. One of the most common ways to detect the chakras is to use a pendulum. The pendulum consists of a stone, a piece of wood, or some other object suspended on a string. It is held about a half inch above the chakra position on the body. The object will pick up the spin of the chakra and reveal details about the chakra's function. When working with an individual to determine what chakra is in need of balancing, the pendulum is an easy method to use. However, when working with yourself, it is also easy to do a simple assessment of your thoughts, emotions, and actions, and pin down the chakras that are out of whack. I have often attempted to check my chakras in the mirror, but it is better to have someone check your chakras for you or to perform your own personal assessment (or both). When I chose my paper and ink colors for my writing experiences, I used my choice of colors as a form of self-assessment. The colors I picked became my study area for the day, and periodically during the day, I would work on balancing, supporting, and focusing on the chakras the colors represented.

Living a balanced life is something many people talk about, and they even attempt it many times, without success. What they fail to realize is that you can't live a balanced life starting from an imbalanced place. If our minds are imbalanced, it is unrealistic to believe we can make wise choices for ourselves. If our body is physically ill, it is unrealistic to believe that we can be energetic and lively. If our spirit is imbalanced, there is no way we can feel a consistent connection with our creator or other individuals. What we truly have to do is "stop, drop, and roll!" We have to put the fire out or just stop our madness right then and there. We may not be able to change things immediately, but stopping to reassess where we currently are out helps open up a more level playing field for ourselves. When the playing field is level, we can take a more balanced stance and focus on the task or events more clearly. Have you ever stood on a scale and had a difficult time weighing yourself? You push the weight from one end to the next as you attempt to gauge your current weight. After you push the balance back and forth a few times, you get closer and closer to pinning down your actual weight. The next time you weigh yourself, it is so much easier because you have an idea of how much you weigh and where the balance needs to go (provided you have not gained or lost a significant amount of weight).

Keeping the chakras balanced allows us to live the balanced life we thought we could only dream about. Living a balanced life is achievable. The catch is, we have to constantly work to maintain that balance. Things may go well at work and at home for a period of time, but something definitely will come along to disrupt the harmony. Your harmony need not be disrupted permanently, nor should you feel bad about being thrown off kilter. Simply identify the area of disruption, readjust yourself, and achieve balance once more. When our chakras are balanced, we can identify our middle ground and get their STAT. The benefits we gain from keeping our chakras balanced are endless and can be seen on many levels—body, mind, and spirit. Some of these benefits are listed below.

Physical Benefits of Having Balanced Chakras

- Keeps us vibrant and youthful
- Helps cleanse the body
- Improves the immune system's function
- Helps oxygenate the body
- Improves metabolism

Mental Benefits of Having Balanced Chakras

- Improves sleeping
- Provides inner peace and clarity
- Decreases anxiety
- Decreases stress
- Decreases depression
- Improves mental stamina

Spiritual Benefits of Having Balanced Chakras

- Improves attention span
- Improves memory
- Decreases negative self-talk
- Provides sense of purpose

- Provides clarity and inner peace
- Promotes confidence in one's outlook on life

There are seven chakras, and each has a specific role and function in the body. When we come into the world, our chakras begin to absorb the energy of our life's experiences. The absorption of that energy can create health or illness, depending on the way in which we allow our experiences to impact us. The chakra is a lens that allows us to see and act in the world in many different ways. If the lens is cloudy or defected, we will function in a cloudy or defected way. If the lens is clear, we can function with clarity and harmony. The ultimate goal is to maximize our highest potential.

Terms Related to Chakras

Aura – The energy field that surrounds the human physical body, made up of several energy bodies.

Biofield – The body's subtle energy field.

Electromagnetic field – The force field that relates to charges of electricity in motion.

Description: Chakra 1 – Staying Alive

Sanskrit name: Muladhara (root or support)

Location: Base of spine, perineum

Purpose: Survival, foundation, grounding, and security

Issues: Work, home, family, health, structure, finances, trust, nourishment, and security

Element: Earth

Color: Red

Orientation: Self-preservation

Associated body parts: Bones, skeletal structure, and teeth

Sensory function: Smell

Description of chakra: Four-petaled flower

Correlation to glands: Adrenal glands and suprarenal glands

Correlation to parts of body: Teeth, nails, blood formation, sciatic nerve, and digestion

Correlation to mental/emotional issues:

Healthy: Work, home, family, health, structure, finances, trust, nourishment, and security

Unhealthy: Fatigue, scattered attention

Correlation to physical issues:

Healthy: Strong teeth, nails, bones, and regular bowel patterns

Unhealthy: Digestive issues, hemorrhoids, irregular bowel patterns (constipation), back pain, sciatica, varicose veins, allergies and reactions, and osteoporosis

Figure 6-2 illustrates the four-petaled flower.

The first chakra relates to our need for survival and to have our needs met. If our basic needs are not met, it is hard to pursue the more spiritual things in life. With a balanced first chakra, we can make sure we get the resources we need to carry out our roles. We are always finding ways to make things work. When we are balanced in this area, we exhibit the following characteristics:

- Groundedness
- Physical health
- Comfortable with body image
- Safe and secure
- Steadfast and solid

Figure 6-2   Chakra 1.

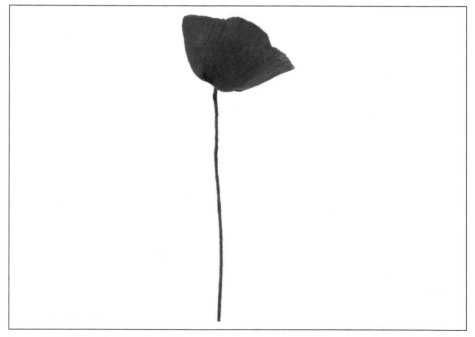

Source: © Keren-S/ShutterStock, Inc.

- Prosperous and abundant
- Inner stillness
- Present in the NOW

Description: Chakra 2 – The Pleasure Principle

Sanskrit name: Svadhisthana (one's own place)

Location: Sacral area, lower back, genitals, and hips

Purpose: Movement

Issues: Sexuality and emotion

Element: Water

Color: Orange

Orientation: Self-gratification

Associated body parts: Sex organs, prostate, and womb

Sensory function: taste

Description of chakra: Six-petaled flower

Correlation to glands: Ovaries and testicles

Correlation to parts of body: Sacral and pelvic region, circulatory, lymphatic system, and urinal and semen flow.

Correlation to mental/emotional issues:

Healthy: Emotions and sexuality

Unhealthy: Sexual imbalance, emotional instability, and aloneness

Correlation to physical issues:

Healthy: Healthy ovaries and testicles, prevention of impotence, and decreased menstrual discomfort

Unhealthy: Dysmenorrhea, fibroids, ovarian cysts, inflammation, impotence, bladder issues, sexually transmitted diseases, kidney issues, hip pain, and incontinence

Figure 6-3 illustrates the six-petaled flower.

The ability to enjoy our lives, relationships, and experience pleasure all has to do with the second chakra. When your second chakra is balanced, you can have fun outside of work and not feel like you are cheating. You can relax at home and not feel like you must complete all the tasks on a 20-page to-do list as well. When we are balanced and in harmony, we exhibit the following characteristics:

- Graceful movements
- Flexibility
- Emotional maturity and intelligence

Figure 6-3   Chakra 2.

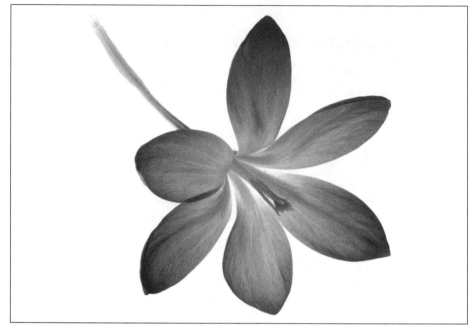

Source: © saied shahin kiya/ShutterStock, Inc.

- Self-nurturing and nurturing of others
- Healthy boundaries
- Passion
- Sexual satisfaction
- Ability to enjoy pleasure

Description: Chakra 3 – The Strive Drive

Sanskrit name: Manipura (lustrous gem)

Location: Solar plexus

Purpose: Energy and will

Issues: Personal power, strength of will, self-mastery, self-esteem, and individuation

Element: Fire

Color: Yellow

Orientation: Self-definition

Associated body parts: Digestive system and muscles

Sensory function: Sight

Description of chakra: Ten-petaled flower

Correlation to glands: Pancreas

Correlation to parts of body: Digestive system and autonomic nervous system

Correlation to mental/emotional issues:

> Healthy: Personal power, strength of will, self-mastery, self-esteem, and individuation

> Unhealthy: Sensitive to criticism, low self-esteem, and controlling

Correlation to physical issues:

> Healthy: Healthy digestive systems, liver, gallbladder, stomach, autonomic nervous system is steady, emotional balance, balanced eating habits

> Unhealthy: Stomach ulcers, gastroesophageal reflux disease, liver issues, spleen issues, gallbladder issues, nerve disorders, eating disorders, gastritis, and jaundice

Figure 6-4 illustrates the 10-petaled flower.

Figure 6-4　Chakra 3.

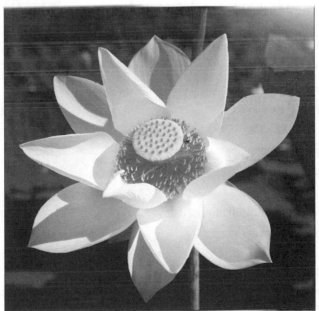

Source: © Khoroshunova Olga/ShutterStock, Inc.

The third chakra represents our will or our core. When this is strong, we can make decisions that are in our best interest. No one can tell you to do something that will jeopardize yourself, your family, your license, or even your self-integrity, because you are strong in who you are. The characteristics of a balanced third chakra are as follows:

- Responsible
- Self-disciplined
- Strong sense of self
- Confident
- Warm
- Energized
- Spontaneous
- Humorous
- Fearless

Description: Chakra 4 – Looking for Love

Sanskrit name: Anahata (unbroken)

Location: Chest and cardiac plexus

Purpose: Love, relationship, and compassion

Issues: Relationship, self-love, and balance

Element: Air

Color: Green

Orientation: Self-acceptance

Associated body parts: Heart, chest, lungs, and circulation

Sensory function: Touch

Description of chakra: 12-petaled flower

Correlation to glands: Thymus

Correlation to physical/mental issues:

    Healthy: Trust issues, codependency, and sadness

    Unhealthy: Relationship, self-love, and balance

Correlation to physical issues:

    Healthy: Balanced respiratory system, immune system, and healthy skin

    Unhealthy: Cardiac issues, cholesterol issues, respiratory infections, allergies, viruses, back pain, costochondritis, shoulder pain, and skin rashes

Figure 6-5   Chakra 4.

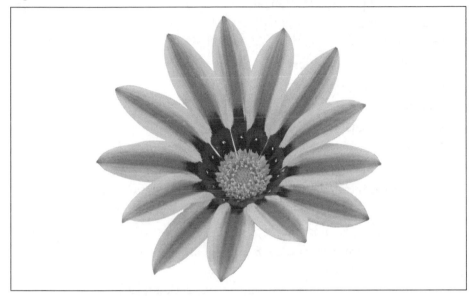

Source: © S1001/ShutterStock, Inc.

Figure 6-5 illustrates the 12-petaled flower.

I sometimes think that songwriters sell the heart a little short, such as when they write songs like "The Heart Is Not So Smart" (by DeBarge). A balanced heart is brilliant! It is when the heart is not in a state of balance that you run into difficulties. Being able to exhibit unconditional love and compassion is a part of this chakra, and it is more challenging than having enemies, because not many people can be completely open to others. A balanced heart chakra exhibits the following characteristics:

- Compassionate and caring
- Empathetic
- Accepting of others
- Self-loving
- Serene
- Grounded
- Satisfied and content

Description: Chakra 5 – Creativity Speaks

Sanskrit name: Visuddha (pure)

Location: Throat

Purpose: Communication and creativity

Issues: Self-expression, speaking one's truth, and listening

Element: Sound

Color: Bright blue

Orientation: Self-expression

Associated body part: Mouth, throat, and ears

Sensory function: Hearing

Description of chakra: 16-petaled flower

Correlation to glands: Thyroid and parathyroid glands

Correlation to mental/emotional issues:

> Healthy: Self-expression, speaking one's truth, and listening
>
> Unhealthy: Perfectionism, writer/artist's block, and unemotional

Correlation to physical issues:

> Healthy: Strong voice, clear breathing, strong vertebrae in the neck, and good hearing
>
> Unhealthy: Throat pain, speech defects, neck issues, shoulder pain, thyroid issues, and dental and periodontal issues

Figure 6-6 illustrates the 18-petaled flower.

The fifth chakra relates to speaking from a place of knowing, as well as to the ability to listen. With these skills, creativity can emerge and many forms of artistic expression can come forward. Having a balanced fifth chakra allows us to show the following qualities:

- Clear communication with others
- Resonant, full voice
- Good listener
- Timing and rhythm
- Creative living

Description: Chakra 6 – To Infinity and Beyond

Sanskrit name: Ajna (perceive and command)

Location: Brow

Purpose: Seeing, intuition, and insight

Issues: Intuition, clarity, vision, and imagination

Element: Light

Color: Indigo

Figure 6-6   Chakra 5.

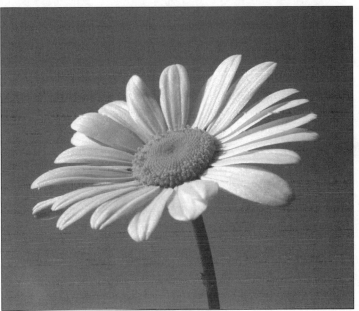

Source: © Stephen Aaron Rees/ShutterStock, Inc.

Orientation: Self-reflection

Associated body part: Eyes and base of skull

Sensory function: Sixth sense

Description of chakra: Two-petaled flower

Correlation to glands: Pituitary gland

Correlation to mental/emotional issues:

> Healthy: Intuition, clarity, vision, and imagination

> Unhealthy: Nightmares, hallucinations, and disabilities

Correlation to physical issues:

> Healthy: Mental clarity, intelligence, concentration, and attention

> Unhealthy: Migraines, headaches, eye issues, brain issues, sinus issues, nerve disorders, mental illness, and mental disability

Figure 6-7 illustrates the two-petaled flower.

The sixth chakra brings us into the more mental and spiritual levels, which give us different challenges for learning. Having the ability to gather information

Figure 6-7   Chakra 6.

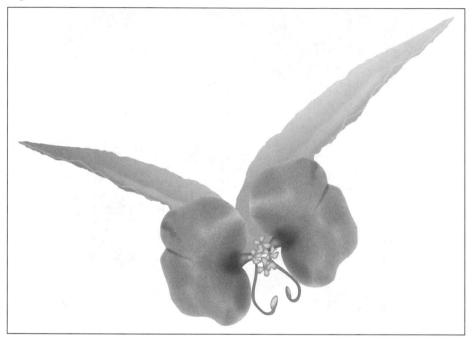

from our surroundings, our experiences, and the unlimited knowledge available to us from the universe gives us quite an opportunity to learn. Nurses have a great sense of intuition because they are able to use their minds, hearts, and experiences to key into the possibilities that usually end up occurring. There is nothing magical about it, because it is something that is natural when we are balanced and in tune with our third eye. The characteristics of this chakra are as follows:

- Intuitive
- Insightful
- Imaginative
- Memory recall
- Dream recall
- Imagery skills
- Visionary

Description: Chakra 7 – The Wisdom of the Infinite

Sanskrit name: Sahasrara (1000-fold)

Location: Crown of head and cerebral cortex

Purpose: Pure awareness, understanding, and unity with the divine

Issues: Spiritual connection, understanding, and intelligence

Element: Thought and consciousness

Color: Violet or white

Orientation: Self-knowledge

Associated body part: Upper skull, cerebral, cortex, and skin

Sensory function: Cosmic awareness

Description of chakra: 1000-petaled lotus flower

Correlation to glands: Pineal gland

Correlation to parts of body: Cerebrum and entire being

Correlation to mental/emotional issues:

> Healthy: Spiritual connection, understanding, and intelligence

> Unhealthy: Depression, obsessive behaviors, and confusion

Correlation to physical issues:

> Healthy: Longevity

> Unhealthy: Headaches, immune deficiency, nervousness, mental illness, confusion, sleep issues, paralysis, and multiple sclerosis

Figure 6-8 illustrates the 1000-petaled flower.

The seventh chakra connects us to the infinite, our higher guidance, our inner wisdom, etc. There are so many different ways to express the connection that links us to God and to each other. Many yogis and wise beings, such as Jesus and Buddha, have walked this path and left an impression on us for life. The characteristics of this chakra are as follows:

- Spiritually connected
- Wise
- Presence
- Intelligent
- Open-minded
- Assimilative and analytical
- Mastery

CHAKRA SELF-CARE PRACTICES

Clearing the Chakras

Clearing the chakras simply means ridding the chakras of energetic debris that may be throwing off the normal clockwise spin. Clearing the chakras establishes

Figure 6-8   Chakra 7.

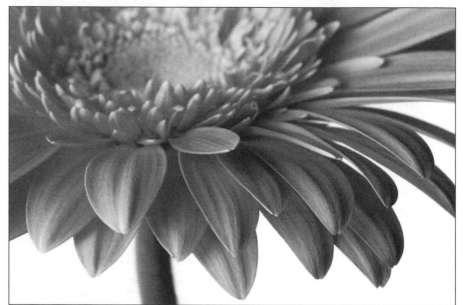

Source: © Tischenko Irina/ShutterStock, Inc.

balance and reestablishes the normal clockwise flow. This can be achieved in many creative ways, including meditation, visualization, aromatherapy, color therapy, music therapy, and what I call "chakra talk."

Meditation

Meditation is an excellent way to clear the chakras and establish balance in the body. Anodea Judith has produced many meditation CDs and books that will walk you through the chakra-balancing experience. I would definitely advise you to invest in her information as a resource. Meditation can be as simple or complex as you make it, but simplicity always works best for me. After I have determined what chakra is in need of support, I meditate on it. If more than one chakra is off, I will meditate on each chakra individually during the day, or on an entire balanced chakra system. There is no right or wrong way to bring harmony to yourself. These exercises are meant to be modified and should be used as a springboard for your own personal creativity. Use them and modify them to suit your own personal needs.

Exercise

Find a comfortable place to sit—on a chair, a couch, or a pillow on the floor. Place your hands in your lap, with palms facing upward. Elevate your gaze slightly and close your eyes. Allow your breath to flow in, as your belly fills. Allow your breath to flow out, as your belly deflates. Repeat this process and continue to breathe in a normal fashion. Pick the chakra that you want to support and meditate on it. As other thoughts come your way, gently release those thoughts and return back to the chakra you are meditating on. It's as simple as that!

Visualization to Clear the Chakras

Visualization is a lot like meditation, except that you are picturing the process of balancing the chakras in your mind's eye. When you can visualize something, it is as good as done, because your brain does not notice the difference. With visualization, you can go through the process of clearing each chakra and restoring balance to your body, mind, and spirit.

Exercise

Find a comfortable place to sit or lie down, with your spine straight. Allow your body to be comfortable and relaxed as you take deep, slow breaths in through the mouth and out through the nose. See the aura that surrounds your entire body. Gently take your hands and place them at the center of the aura directly above your head. Take both your hands and part the aura directly down the center, allowing half of the aura to gently fall to one side of your body and the other half to gently fall to the other side.

Imagine your chakras lying open and exposed. You can see every one of them. Cover yourself in light and love as they come from heaven and saturate your exposed body. Visualize the light filling your body, as it waits ready to support you in balancing each of your chakras.

We begin with the root chakra first. Imagine your hand moving the chakra counterclockwise, as if you were removing a lid from a jar. Direct the love and light to that chakra to fill it up to the brim. Take your imaginary hand and begin a clockwise motion, as if you were putting the lid back on the jar.

Next, visualize your sacral chakra. Imagine your hand moving the chakra counterclockwise, as if you were removing a lid from a jar. Direct the love and light to that chakra to fill it up to the brim. Take your imaginary hand and begin a clockwise motion, as if you were putting the lid back on a jar.

Next, visualize your solar plexus chakra. Imagine your hand moving the chakra counterclockwise, as if you were removing a lid from a jar. Direct the love and light to that chakra to fill it up to the brim. Take your imaginary hand and begin a clockwise motion, as if you were putting the lid back on the jar.

Next, visualize your heart chakra. Imagine your imaginary hand moving the chakra counterclockwise, as if you were removing a lid from a jar. Direct the love and light to that chakra to fill it up to the brim. Take your imaginary hand and begin a clockwise motion, as if you were putting the lid back on the jar.

Next, visualize your throat chakra. See your hand moving the chakra counterclockwise, as if you were removing a lid from a jar. Direct the love and light to that chakra to fill it up to the brim. Take your imaginary hand and begin a clockwise motion, as if you were putting the lid back on the jar.

Next, visualize your brow chakra. Imagine your etheric hand moving the chakra counterclockwise, as if you were removing a lid from a jar. Direct the love and light to that chakra to fill it up to the brim. Take your etheric hand and begin a clockwise motion, as if you were putting the lid back on the jar.

Next, visualize your crown chakra. Imagine your hand moving the chakra counterclockwise, as if you were removing a lid from a jar. Direct the love and light to that chakra to fill it up to the brim. Visualize taking your hand and beginning a clockwise motion, as if you were putting the lid back on the jar. Visualize taking your hand and brushing away any debris that has been released from the balancing of the chakras. Allow the love and light to seal up any leaks in the body (mental, spiritual, or physical). Use your hands to gather the aura back together. Seal it with love and light. Share your prayer of gratitude for the experience, the awareness, and the wisdom to self-heal. Take three nice deep, clearing breaths, and allow your body to awaken feeling refreshed, invigorated, and totally balanced within.

Essential Oils for Clearing

Aromatherapy is very beneficial for balancing the chakra system of the body. Each essential oil has a function that supports certain chakras and allows normalcy to return. Aromas can draw us to others just as quickly as they can repel us. The sense of smell stimulates our emotions and connects us to places that bring back memories from the deepest parts of our minds.

Many essential oils are available to us through holistic venues. These oils are very concentrated and should not be placed directly on your skin. Usually, essential oils for direct application are mixed with a base oil, which dilutes the concentration of the oil and allows you to use it on your skin without causing severe irritation. Good base oils include olive oil, canola oil, and grapeseed oil, among others.

Exercise 1

Determine which chakra or chakras are in need of your attention. Select an essential oil from Table 6-1 that corresponds with the chakra(s) that are in need. If

Table 6-1   Chakra Essential Oil and Color Table

Chakras	Essential Oil Suggestions	Corresponding Chakra Colors
1st Chakra	Cedarwood, Sandalwood, Cypress	Red
2nd Chakra	Clary Sage, Patchouli, Anise	Orange
3rd Chakra	Rosemary, Juniper, Peppermint	Yellow
4th Chakra	Rose, Ylang-Ylang, Eucalyptus	Green
5th Chakra	Tea-Tree Oil, Neroli, Frankincense	Blue
6th Chakra	Jasmine, Elemi, Melissa	Indigo
7th Chakra	Vetiver, Myrhh, Frankincense	Violet/Purple

you have a little bottle (preferably amber-colored, because light tends to break down the oil), place a milliliter of base oil in the bottle. Place a few drops of each essential oil into the bottle for each chakra you are working on. This creates a blend that you can use to balance your chakras throughout the day. Enjoy the benefits of the aroma. Use the mixture periodically during the day on your hands and body. (If you are new to oils and need to make a blend, do not mix them together in one bottle initially. If you find you have a sensitivity to an essential oil, you will need to know which oil is causing the sensitivity.) Once you have experienced each oil and determined that you have no sensitivities, you can create a blend and use it regularly.

Exercise 2

Determine which chakra requires your attention. Select an essensial oil from Table 6-1 that corresponds with the chakra(s) that are in need. Place a few drops of the essential oil on a tissue and place it in your pocket. At given periods throughout the day, take out the tissue and enjoy the aroma you have selected. Take note of how you feel and how the smell impacts your thinking and your actions. Write about your experiences.

Color Therapy

Each chakra is associated with a different color in the rainbow. We subconsciously seek out the colors we need to establish balance within us. The colors we are drawn to may also be those that are strongest in our auric field.

Exercise 1

Determine the chakra that needs your support. Select a corresponding color(s) from Table 6-1 that corresponds with the color(s) of the chakra(s) that are in need. Look in your closet and pick out an outfit with the colors you need to balance and harmonize yourself. If your outfit doesn't yield the most perfect combination of colors, don't forget that you can wear colored undergarments too! You can also use colored pieces of paper, cards, and jewelry to balance your chakras. Note the way you feel wearing the colors and how your day is impacted each time you look at them. Record your experiences in your journal.

Exercise 2

You are never too old to color. Go to your local store and purchase a set of crayons and a coloring book, and use the colors that are speaking to you. Color to your heart's content and observe the changes in your mood. Record your impressions of the colors you chose, and how you feel the coloring impacted your overall balance.

Music Therapy

Music is available that has been created for the sole purpose of balancing the chakras.

Listening to music has very calming and therapeutic effects that can help restore overall balance to the body.

Exercise

Search online for chakra music, or do a little shopping at your local music store and see what you can come up with. A good Web site is Pandora (www.pandora.com), and of course you can download iTunes (if you have an iPod) for a fee from the iTunes site. You can create your own chakra-balancing soundtrack to help you harmonize your body, mind, and spirit.

Chakra Talk

"Chakra talk" is something that I do when I'm feeling out of balance and cannot immediately meditate, visualize, or listen to a relaxation tape on the spot. Because I spend a lot of time in my car, visiting patients' homes throughout the day, I often use that time to "talk to my chakras," which basically means that I direct them to correct themselves for my highest good. By the time I've reached my destination, my chakras have been given the pep talk they need, and I'm beginning to receive the balance I deserve.

Hands-On Ritual for Clearing

This ritual is very similar to the visualization exercise, but is done with a partner. If you are reading this book as part of a group, pick a partner and make a date to balance your chakras.

Exercise

Set the intention that your partner's chakras will be balanced for his or her highest good. Make your partner as comfortable as you can, on a chair or a massage table (a steady table or bed will do). Encourage them to allow their body to be comfortable and relaxed while he or she takes in deep, slow breaths in through the mouth and out through the nose. You may not see the aura that surrounds their entire body, but go through the motions and peel the aura down like a banana.

Gently take your hands and place them at the center of the aura directly above your partner's head. Take both of your hands and part the aura directly down the center, allowing half of the aura to gently fall to one side of their body and the other half to gently fall to the other side. Imagine their chakras lying open and exposed. You may not be able to see the chakras aligning the spinal cord, but that is okay.

Cover yourself and your partner in light and love as it shines from heaven and saturate your partner's exposed body and chakra system. Visualize the light filling his or her body, as it waits ready to support you in balancing each chakra. We begin with the root chakra first. Take your hand and begin moving the chakra counterclockwise, as if you were removing a lid from a jar. Direct the love and light to that chakra to fill it up to the brim. Take your hand and begin a clockwise motion, as if you were putting the lid back on the jar.

Next, focus on the sacral chakra. Imagine your hand moving the chakra counterclockwise, as if you were removing a lid from a jar. Direct the love and light to that chakra to fill it up to the brim. Take your hand and begin a clockwise motion, as if you were putting the lid back on the jar.

Next, focus on their solar plexus chakra. Imagine your hand moving the chakra counterclockwise, as if you were removing a lid from a jar. Direct the love and light to that chakra to fill it up to the brim. Take your hand and begin a clockwise motion, as if you were putting the lid back on the jar.

Next, focus on the heart chakra. Imagine your hand moving the chakra counterclockwise, as if you were removing a lid from a jar. Direct the love and light to that chakra to fill it up to the brim. Take your hand and begin a clockwise motion, as if you were putting the lid back on the jar.

Next, focus on the throat chakra. Imagine your hand moving the chakra counterclockwise, as if you were removing a lid from a jar. Direct the love and light to that chakra to fill it up to the brim. Take your hand and begin a clockwise motion, as if you were putting the lid back on the jar.

Next, focus on the brow chakra. Imagine your hand moving the chakra counterclockwise, as if you were removing a lid from a jar. Direct the love and light to that chakra to fill it up to the brim. Take your hand and begin a clockwise motion, as if you were putting the lid back on the jar.

Next, focus on the crown chakra. Imagine your hand moving the chakra counter-clockwise, as if you were removing a lid from a jar. Direct the love and light to that chakra to fill it up to the brim. Take your hand and begin a clockwise motion, as if you were putting the lid back on the jar. Take your hand and brush away any debris that has been released from the balancing of your partner's chakras. Allow the love and light to seal up any leaks in his or her body (mental, spiritual, or physical). With your hands, gather the aura back together. Seal it with love and light. Share your prayer of gratitude for the experience, the awareness, and the wisdom to help others to heal. Encourage your partner to begin taking nice deep, clearing breaths while he or she allows his or her body to awaken refreshed, invigorated, and totally balanced within.

Take a 15-minute break and allow your partner to record his or her experience, drink some water, and get grounded. Switch places and take your turn getting your chakras balanced. Enjoy the experience and describe it in your journal.

EXPERIENCING CHAKRA-BALANCING AS A CLIENT

Selecting a Chakra Therapist

A chakra-balancing session is similar in many ways to a Reiki or Healing Touch treatment. I believe this is because those modalities have specific practices that also incorporate chakra balancing. The Chakra Therapist or practitioner prepares the same way a Reiki or Healing Touch Practitioner would prepare for a regular healing session, says a prayer of intention, opens the aura, balances the chakras, closes the aura, and sweeps any debris that may be left in the field. You can find a chakra-balancing therapist online, through holistic listings, or in holistic news-papers in your area.

Pricing for Sessions

The price for a session ranges from $30 to $65 an hour.

Duration of Sessions

The sessions range in duration from 30 minutes to 1 hour.

What to Expect From a Session

The client should feel relaxed and feel very rested. I balanced my eldest daughter's chakras when she was about 14 years of age. When I was done, I asked her how she enjoyed the session. She said, "It's weird, Mommy, like I like my sister more now." That's not really what I was expecting, but I gathered that she had a stronger sense of love for her sister and that I must have done something special with her heart chakra.

FURTHER STUDIES IN THE CHAKRA SYSTEM

Chakra Training

Many years ago, I completed a chakra program offered by the Reiki Blessings Academy, which is still in existence. The chakra-balancing therapy course at Reiki Blessings Academy certifies you to balance chakras for family, friends, and clients. You can visit www.reikiblessings.com for more information regarding the program. When I took the class (by correspondence), I was required to do homework, obtain essential oils and stones, examine case studies, and take a test at the end. It was fun and not too demanding, and gave me a basic introduction to chakras. The price for the class was about $100. Another program is sponsored by Anodea Judith, through Sacred Centers. This is a general certificate program that is open to anyone and has no prerequisites. Sacred Centers also offers a professional program that consists of four different tracts: Sacred Centers Teacher (to teach the curriculum), Chakra Therapist (to incorporate chakra information into the clinical setting), Chakrassage (to incorporate chakra work into energetic modalities), and Sacred Centers Coaching (to help clients use the chakra model to look at their problems and determine how they are relating to their issues and how they can create tools to deal with those issues in healing ways). These are not correspondence courses. The Sacred Centers Web site (www.sacredcenters.com) has detailed information and brochures for downloading. I encourage you to visit the site and explore more if you desire.

Associations

To my knowledge, there are no associations related to chakra therapy, but there are many books and resources that can help you in your studies. You can always surf the Web for information. Not all the information on the Web is beneficial, however. Use your best judgment and consult with people you know in or outside your area.

REFERENCES

Bruyere, R. L. (1994). *Wheels of light*. New York: Fireside Publishing.

Judith, A. (2003). *Wheels of life*. St. Paul, MN: Llewellyn Publications.

Koopsen, C., & Young, C. (2009). *Integrative health*. Sudbury, MA: Jones & Bartlett.

SUGGESTED READING LIST

Fallon, S. (2001). *Nourishing traditions*. Washington, DC: New Trends Publishing.

Libster, M. (2002). *Delmar's integrative herb guide for nurses*. Albany, NY: Delmar Publishing Company.

CHAPTER 7

Introduction to Kundalini Yoga

RACHEL Y. HILL

"Kundalini yoga is uncoiling yourself to find your potential and your vitality and to reach for your virtues. There is nothing from outside. Try to understand that. All is in you. You are the storehouse of your totality."

—YOGI BHAJAN

MY PERSONAL STORY

I kept yoga on my list of "things to do and/or learn" for quite some time. I finally took my first yoga class at the YMCA, after 8 years of wondering what a yoga class would really be like. The class was an enjoyable experience, but I didn't practice yoga again until a year later. Why had I kept yoga on my list for so long? Half of my mind would like to think that the time was just not right then (as a nurse and mother, I was always so very busy). The other half of me believes that I was very much fixated on the images of yogis and instructors (on fancy DVD covers in incredibly flexible poses, with incredibly lean bodies) who had been teaching yoga for 50 years and didn't look a day over 25. I think I was a little intimidated by the possibility of making a fool of myself. In the meantime, while I was working with my own self-limitations, I purchased a DVD to practice yoga at home in private. I wanted to at least work up to a level of competence before my public re-debut as a student. I picked a DVD pretty much at random from the store shelf, but once I put it in the DVD player and listened to the instructor's initial comments, I knew I had picked the right one. The instructor was probably in her mid- to late 40s, but she said that she began studying yoga when she was about 35. That encouraged me. She went on to say that she could not even touch her toes when she took her first class! I gave a loud "yes!" Not because I was so happy she was in just as bad a shape as I was, but because there was hope for me to begin studies in yoga. She helped me realize that I didn't have to be perfect. All I really needed was the heart to go beyond my physical limitations.

I was first introduced to Kundalini yoga exercises at a school where I studied metaphysics, but I didn't learn anything in depth at that time. Kundalini is the energy that rests dormant in our root chakra or the base of our spine, and is released and coils upward with spiritual awakening. I decided I would start with Kundalini, because it is more meditative. I wanted the physical aspects of exercise, but I also wanted a meditative, spiritual practice. There was an ashram in my area, which was very exciting for me. When I arrived, I discovered that one of the teachers was a social worker and our paths had crossed many times in our lines of work. The teachers were very kind and thoroughly explained the various things that I might experience during my session. Once I began the session, I had a series of thoughts ranging from "I want to go home!" to "Wow, this is bliss!" I experienced many things I had never experienced before in any form of meditation or exercises I had ever done. The only difference was that it was all combined!

In my third or fourth class, my yoga teacher gave me a brochure for the Kundalini Yoga Teacher Training Program. I thought that becoming a yoga teacher with my current knowledge base would be like becoming a nurse after only taking a basic nursing-skills class. This would (and should never) happen in the real world! I knew I wanted to study Kundalini yoga more, but I politely turned down the offer and said that I would revisit the idea next year, after I had more practice. I wasn't feeling qualified to teach a yoga class for anyone, anytime, anywhere. My teacher was very straightforward and told me it didn't matter how many classes I took. He went on to share a quote with me from the master who brought Kundalini yoga to the west: Karta Purkh would often tell me from the words of Yogi Bhajan, "If you want to learn something, read about it. If you want to understand something, write about it. If you want to master something, teach it." Needless to say, I began the Kundalini yoga teacher training course over the next year, and deepened my understanding of yoga practices.

HISTORY OF KUNDALINI YOGA

Kundalini yoga is a science that has been around for thousands of years and is known as the "mother of all yogas." During the golden ages or a time of great enlightenment, yoga was openly practiced and taught. It was after this age that many schools of yoga developed from the various transitions that were taking place. Devotees wanted to preserve the science as best they could. Persecution and natural disasters caused the yogis to disperse to different geographical areas. For safety reasons, they had to be very selective about whom they would choose to teach Kundalini yoga. In some instances, the dispersal of the yogis led to the development of various forms of yoga. Eventually, there were very few yogis who knew the complete teachings of Kundalini yoga. This ancient science was passed down orally from Masters to dedicated students. Students who desired to learn Kundalini yoga had to serve their Master and prove their dedication, self-discipline, and humility before the teacher would even consider taking them on as a student. This also helped protect the science from those who might want to manipulate it for selfish purposes. Much power comes from the awareness of Kundalini; therefore, it couldn't be entrusted to just anyone.

Yogi Bhajan (also called Harbhajan Singh Puri) was born a prince more than 70 years ago. It was prophesied that he was destined for greatness and would change the lives of millions. His family was very wealthy and owned entire villages in what is now Pakistan. Growing up, his birthdays were celebrations that the family used to share its wealth with the poor. His parents would give his body weight in gold, copper, and silver, or seven times his weight in grain. Through this, he learned about sharing with others.

Yogi Bhajan was educated in an all-girls Catholic school and became a master of Kundalini yoga in India at the age of 16 years. He went on to graduate from college, serve in the military, start a family, and work as an officer in Customs, until an opportunity presented itself that changed his life and brought Kundalini yoga to the west. Yogi Bhajan was invited to teach Kundalini yoga in Canada at the University of Toronto. He accepted the offer in September of 1968. Yogi Bhajan wanted to share yoga with Americans and other Europeans because he believed many of them were exploited in their journeys to learn yoga in India. Yogi Bhajan was about empowering others to find their own way, with the proper tools for their own spiritual path. When he arrived in Canada, however, he discovered that the person who had invited him had been killed in an accident, and his luggage had been lost. With no luggage and only a few dollars in his pocket, he realized that his plans were suddenly changed.

Yogi Bhajan then received an invitation from a friend in Los Angeles to spend the weekend. He met so many young people who were seeking a spiritual path that he decided to act on that energy and help them to meet their destiny through the spiritual path of yoga. He decided to stay and help them usher in the "Aquarian Age" through his yogic teachings of the Kundalini Science. He stayed in Los Angeles for a while and then moved to New Mexico, where the Kundalini yoga headquarters (3HO) was established. Yogi Bhajan had a great following, but never intended to have a group of disciples. He wanted to train teachers and was quick to tell everyone that this was his ultimate goal. He encouraged others to "learn and teach what you have learned to others." Yogi Bhajan broke the secrecy of the yoga tradition and helped many people who might otherwise have turned to a life of drugs and, ultimately, death, by sharing ways to support the physical body, health, and wellness with yoga. Yogi Bhajan was a master of many things, aside from Kundalini yoga, all of which have had an impact on what he has been able to teach others. From Ayurvedic healing to Hatha yoga and recipes for cooking, health remedies, and cleansing, his knowledge has influenced many people.

CONCEPT OF KUNDALINI YOGA

The concept of Kundalini yoga, in a nutshell, is to support individuals in expanding self-awareness and promoting self-healing. Kundalini yoga practices support the physical body with exercises that help support the immune system, organ function, cleansing of the body, and healthy nerve function. In Kundalini yoga, the spine is very important because the flexibility of the spine is the true determinant of youthfulness, as well as the vehicle by which the Kundalini energy ascends and descends. In my first Kundalini yoga class, my teacher, Karta Purkh, would frequently remind us that if we kept our spine flexible, we would never get old. I knew he didn't mean that we would never age, but that we would remain more youthful and grow older much more gracefully.

Kundalini yoga practices also support the negative experiences we have every day, such as fear, anger, grief, and doubt. There are many opportunities throughout the day when we can use yoga to help us face a difficult situation. Last but not least, there are yogic exercises that connect us with our divine source of life, through meditation and prayer. All these practices impact all aspects of our health, allowing us to live up to our fullest potential. Yoga is "a complete science that combines posture (asana), movement, breath work (pranayama), chanting (mantra) and meditation into powerful sets called Kriyas (sequenced sets of exercises) that target specific benefits" (http://www.yogasimran.com). Kundalini yoga is a combination of the tools mentioned above that allows us to find balance within ourselves and in our outer worlds.

Kundalini yoga appealed to me as healthcare provider because every single activity we do in Kundalini yoga is associated with a health benefit of some type. I am always thinking of yogic prescriptions to share with people whose complaints have not been resolved by their healthcare practitioners. Kundalini yoga is focused toward healthy function of the physical body, mental and emotional wellness, and our highest connections with others and our Creator. Not only are these practices excellent for patients, they can also help you to rejuvenate your own body at a moment's notice. These tools are necessary when you are faced with the negativity of job settings, fatigue from a long shift, or even the continuous need nurses have to filter grief, fear, pain, and other strong emotions that can be wearing on the mind. The majority of nurses are now older than the age of 50, and the different exercises Kundalini offers can help keep those nurses more agile, charged, and moving toward retirement gracefully. Kundalini yoga is yet another tool that can bring the restoration we need to maintain harmony in our thinking and cope with stressful situations. With practice, we can learn to become efficient in caring for ourselves and our patients and creating harmony in the healthcare setting, which is very much needed. Kundalini yoga, as well as other forms of yoga, can help us accommodate changes that we might not be able to otherwise.

Terms Related to Kundalini Yoga

Adi mantra – Tuning in before a yoga set or meditation. This mantra is chanted at the beginning of each yoga session to connect us to the divine teacher we have inside. We are able to connect to our yogic lineage through this mantra and tap into the highest guidance, energy, and inspiration. The Adi mantra is "Ong Namo Guru Dev Namo," which means "I call on the infinite creative consciousness."

Asanas – Consciously taken positions that affect an individual's awareness, emotions, and reflexes.

Bhandas – Contractions of the muscle that direct the flow of psychic energy and change the blood circulation, nerve pressure, and cerebral spinal fluid flow.

Kriya – A set of exercises that are used to achieve specific benefits in an individual.

Gyan Mudra – Touching the tip of the index finger to the tip of the thumb in a meditative hand position to achieve balance and expansion.

Kundalini ("coiled serpent") – The energy that rests dormant in the root chakra but is released by spiritual experience.

Mantras – "Man" means mind, and "tra" means to tune the vibration. Mantras are sounds that tune and manage the vibration of the mind, impacting a person's consciousness.

Meditation – Stilling the mind by concentrating on an object or thought and achieving a state of awareness of self-growth and higher consciousness.

Mudras – Finger positions that allow us to connect with the body and the mind, impacting the body's energy system.

Pranayama – Regulated breathing exercises used to achieve a specific purpose within the body.

Sadhana – The practice of performing spiritual exercises, including yoga, meditation, and mantras, every day (usually early in the morning).

Sat Nam – Also called the Bij Mantra, meaning "truth is your identity; God's name is truth." This mantra reinforces our divine consciousness.

Kundalini Yoga Class for Self-Care

Pranayam Exercise – Sitali Pranayama

The Sitali Pranayam is a breathing exercise that helps build strength and increase vitality (Fig. 7-1). It has a very cooling impact as well as a cleansing effect on the body. The tongue may taste bitter initially, but eventually it will taste sweet.

1. Sit in an easy pose or in Indian style with the spine straight.
2. Curl your tongue into a "U" shape.
3. Inhale through your curled tongue and exhale through the mouth.
4. Do this for 3 minutes or 26 times in the morning and/or evening.
5. Do this for a week and record your experiences or impressions in your journal.

Figure 7-1   Sitali pranayam.

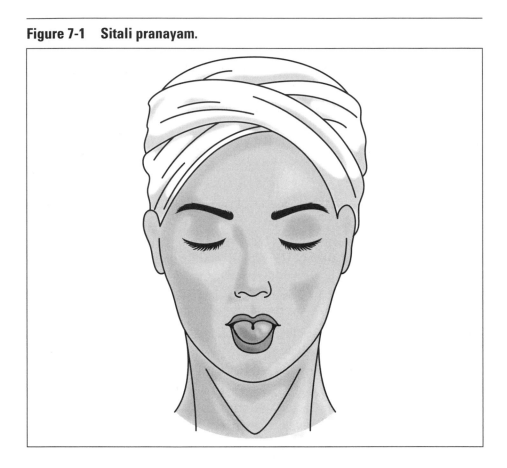

Repeating this exercise 108 times creates a very deep meditation and healing experience for the physical body and the digestive tract (Bhajan, 2003).

Meditation for Concentration in Action

This meditation is taken from a book of meditations and exercises for stress and pressure called the *The Survival Kit*. This meditation is beneficial if you don't have a great deal of experience in meditating. An important component of meditation is concentration. By learning to concentrate, you learn to control the way you react to certain situations. It has the benefit of bringing focus to the most unfocused mind.

1. Sit in the easy pose or Indian style with your spine straight.
2. Take your four fingers of your right hand and feel your pulse in the left wrist. (Place the fingers in a straight line so you can feel the pulsing in your fingertips)

3. Focus your mind at the place where the nose and brows meet, with eyelids slightly closed.
4. As you feel the pulsing, hear the sound "sat naam" in your mind with each beat. This practice can be done for 11 minutes at a time. Continue the practice and eventually you can work up to a longer time period (31 minutes). This practice will help pave the way for you to focus in your meditations.

What to Expect from a Kundalini Yoga Class

Kundalini yoga classes are the best way to experience the energy of creativity that we have talked about and nurture yourself at the same time. It is important to take a yoga class if you have never practiced Kundalini yoga before. It is always better to be under the advice of a teacher before you begin independent practice on your own. There will be positions and breathing techniques that are new to you, and it is good to know that you are doing them correctly and that your body is positioned correctly to prevent physical harm. The class will help you establish the groundwork for safe yoga practices that you can incorporate into your personal study. You have already learned a meditation and a breathing exercise. A Kundalini yoga class is structured as follows:

1. Adi mantra
2. Warm-up
3. Pranayama
4. Kriya
5. Relaxation
6. Meditation
7. Ending prayer
8. Questions and answers

You will experience each of these phases in a Kundalini yoga class. Many teachers will teach the same class for a week, then teach a different class the next week, and so on. In some classes, the teacher will ask the students what they need and will create a yoga set or class based on what the group needs at the time.

Selecting a Class or Teacher

The best way to find a Kundalini yoga class is to contact the 3HO Kundalini Headquarters and ask for a referral to a teacher in your area. The International Kundalini Yoga Teachers Association (IKYTA) can also help you find a teacher in your area. Use your judgment and take the class that feels right to you. Kundalini yoga teachers take their job very seriously. They feel that they have a responsibility for the growth of their students, to encourage them, and help them to reach past their limitations—mentally, spiritually, and physically. There are usually many levels of students in each class, so don't worry about someone staring at you and judging your abilities. The sessions are detailed and give you so much to do that little else will matter to you.

Before you begin classes, you should always consult with your physician. Notify your teacher if you have any muscular/skeletal issues or past injuries. If you are pregnant or on your menstrual cycle, you should ask the teacher for adaptations to the various exercises that involve your abdomen to prevent premature contractions or increased blood flow. The supplies you will need for yoga are usually provided in the class, but many people like to bring their own. These supplies include a yoga mat for performing your Kriya, a pillow to sit on or use to support different poses you might do during your Kriya, and a blanket to cover up with during the relaxation portion of the yoga set. Many people use sheepskin in place of a yoga mat because it's a natural fiber that absorbs energy. Wearing all-natural fibers feel good to your skin and allows it to breathe. No shoes or socks are worn during Kundalini yoga, to allow the feet to breathe and the chakras to be stimulated. The eyes are usually kept closed during yoga class, which helps you conserve energy, visualize, and increase your concentration. Yoga is best done on an empty stomach. For best results and comfort, do not eat within 2 hours of a yoga class. If you need to eat something, eat something very light that will be digested quickly. Most importantly, do the very best you can and keep up your practice if you find that Kundalini yoga is something you enjoy.

Structure of the Class

A typical class might look like this:

Everyone sits in the easy pose with his or her back straight and hands in the prayer pose position. Eyes are closed.

First, everyone tunes in with the Adi mantra ("Ong Namo Guru Dev Namo"; Fig. 7-2)

- Ong: Infinite, creative, and divine, which unites us all
- Namo: I call on the wisdom and the energy and bow to it in reverence
- Guru: Transforming energy from darkness to light
- Dev: The subtle energy within us all
- Namo: I call on that energy and bow in reverence

This mantra connects us to the Golden Chain. The Golden Chain is representative of our yogic lineage. The teacher knows that his or her ego is not at work here. This mantra joins Kundalini teachers to the yogis, masters, and saints who have gone before us on this yogic path. This mantra centers our highest good and helps us to be open to the yoga we experience through practice.

Figure 7-2   Adi mantra.

ADI MANTRA

(OR TUNING IN)

Ong Namo Guru Dev Namo

Ong—ng namo gu—roo

(when pronouncing the r, tap your tongue on the roof of our mouth to make the sound goodu) dayv namo

The way we begin Kundalini Yoga sessions is the way we begin our meditation.

The Adi Mantra means:

I acknowledge the One Creative Consciousness.

I acknowledge the Subtle and Divine Wisdom Within.

Warm-Ups

Neck rolls: Begin by rolling your neck clockwise, inhaling as you roll forward and exhaling as you roll your neck back. Repeat for 2 minutes forward and 2 minutes back.

Shoulder rolls: Begin by rolling the shoulders forward, inhaling as you roll them forward and exhaling as you roll them back. Repeat for 2 minutes forward and 2 minutes back.

Spinal twists: Inhale as you twist from your waist to the right, then twist back to the center. Exhale as you twist from your waist to the left, then twist back to the center. Repeat for 2 minutes forward and 2 minutes back.

Pranayama – Breath of Fire (for energy, focus, and vitality)

The Breath of Fire is a quick, rhythmic, and ongoing breath that sounds like powerful sniffing. You forcefully exhale your breath by rapidly contracting the diaphragm and pulling the navel point toward your spine. When you inhale, this occurs naturally as the diaphragm relaxes and air flows back in without effort. The inhalation and exhalation are of equal duration and usually occur two to three times per second. This breath works great for energizing your body if you are feeling scattered or fatigued. It can be practiced periodically throughout the day, for 30 seconds to 3 minutes, if you need a boost in your energy. Begin with the 3-minute interval.

Steps for breath of fire

1. Sit in the easy pose with your spine straight. Take a deep breath in through your nose, and feel your stomach relaxing outward.
2. Exhale through your nose as you pull your stomach back in.
3. Inhale once more. As you exhale out this time, pull the area above your navel back toward the spine in a pumping motion. (Your exhalation should leave your nose as a forceful blowing out.)
4. Immediately relax the solar plexus and let the air come back in with a sniff. Your inhalation and exhalation should be fluid, with no breaks in between. Continue the pumping motion with the sniff breathing. Begin by focusing on your navel area. As you relax your navel point, you will inhale naturally. Do not overexert yourself during this exercise. If you begin to feel light-headed, dizzy, or short of breath, or to experience pain, relax your breathing pattern. If you are not used to the power of the breath, it can be overwhelming. Practice enables us to become comfortable with what we are able to achieve with the Pranayam.

Kriya (asanas or poses)

A Kriya is a set of Kundalini yoga exercises that are meant to accomplish a specific purpose, such as achieving awareness, a balanced nervous system, endocrine function, etc. Each exercise can range in duration from 1 minute to 1.5, 3, 5, or 7 minutes. The instructor will have a timer and specify the time required for each exercise and also alert you as to how much time you have remaining for each exercise. The Kriya serves to stimulate the organs and systems of the body while bringing a renewal to your overall being.

Kriya for lungs and bloodstream (Kundalini yoga for youth and joy)

Figures 3 and 4 illustrate parts 1 and 2, respectively, of the spinal motion in the Kriya.

This Kriya helps us build stamina and balance the cardiac system. The kidneys, gonads, and adrenals are also balanced in this process. This Kriya is also said to help us to take in oxygen more efficiently and to oxygenate and purify the bloodstream. Illnesses often occur because we do not take oxygen in efficiently.

Figure 7-3 Kriya for lungs and bloodstream part 1.

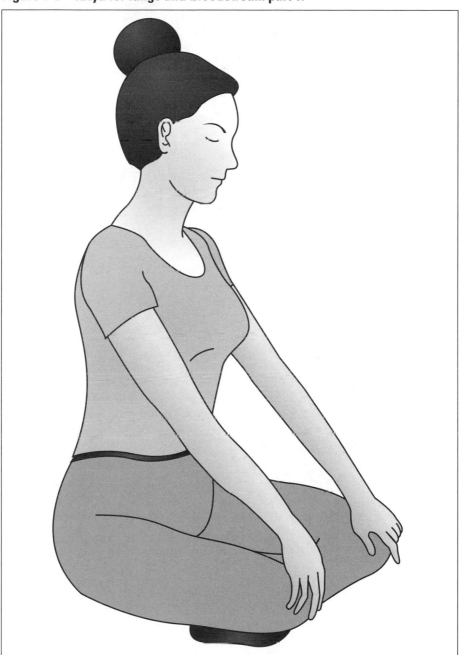

Figure 7-4   Kriya for lungs and bloodstream part 2.

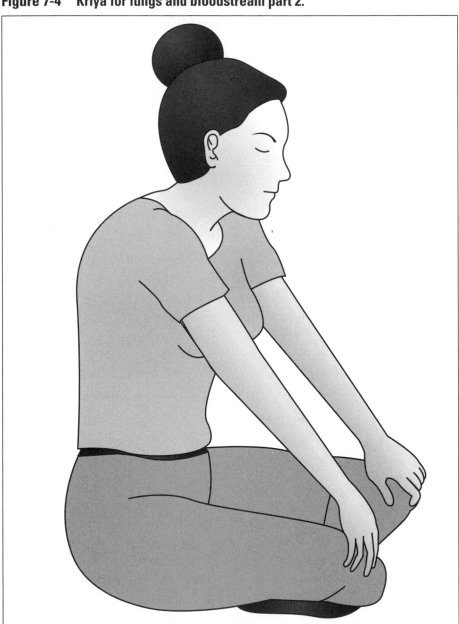

1. Sit in the easy pose your spine straight.
2. Take hold of your knees with hands.
3. Inhale, stretching your rib cage to its maximum capacity (do not sip more air in later, and do not allow air to seep out).
4. Put your tongue behind the upper teeth, where the roof of the mouth meets.
5. Relax the spine and keep the breath held in.
6. Start flexing the spine rapidly until you can no longer hold your breath any longer, then exhale (increase the time you hold your breath gradually to 1 minute).
7. Continue this for 11 minutes, rest, and then continue for 11 minutes more.

Relaxation – lying flat on your back in the corpse pose

In Kundalini yoga, the relaxation phase is the reward for your hard work. You take time to relax so that you can allow the Kriya you have just completed to do its healing and balancing work. This relaxation is often done while listening to music. I enjoy playing various kinds of music with mantras or words that carry powerful meanings, so that the students will be able to absorb the messages and carry them into their lives.

Meditation exercise

Meditation is an important part of a Kundalini yoga class or session. It allows you to turn your attention inward toward yourself. This meditation, which was taken from *The Survival Kit*, is meant to totally recharge you and help with many things, including feelings of depression. This meditation helps support your ability to cope with life as it comes.

1. Sit in the easy pose or in Indian style with your spine straight.
2. Extend your arms out straight in front of you, parallel to the ground.
3. Close your right hand into a fist.
4. Wrap your left fingers around the fist.
5. Allow the base of the palms to touch, with the thumbs close together and pulled straight up.
6. Focus your eyes on your thumbs.
7. Inhale for 5 seconds (but don't hold your breath) and exhale for 5 seconds (hold the breath out for 15 seconds). Eventually you will be able to hold your breath out for 1 minute. You can do this exercise for 3 to 5 minutes to begin with. Eventually, you can work up to a longer time period (11 minutes). Gradually work on building your time, managing your breath. Practice this exercise during your break times, for 1 week (at home and at work).

Ending prayer (this includes a song called the "Sunshine Song" and a prayer or blessing for the class)

The Sunshine Song

May the long time sun shine upon you,
all love surrounds you,
and the pure light within you
guides your way on.
May the long time sun shine upon you,
all love surrounds you,
and the pure light within you
guides your way on, guides your way on, guides your way on.

Bij Mantra or Sat Nam

The Sat Nam is also called the Bij Mantra and means the truth is your identity and God's name is the truth. This mantra reinforces the divinity that we all possess within. This is how we greet each other in Kundalini yoga classes, and it is also used in breathing exercises and Kriyas in yoga class.

Ending prayer

Example: May you have inward peace and share that light with others throughout your week!

Questions and answers

At the end of the class, students are given an opportunity to ask questions about what they felt or experienced during the yoga session.

Benefits of Kundalini Yoga

The benefits of Kundalini yoga have been mentioned throughout the chapter and are not limited to the following list:

- Works on your entire system (nervous, glandular, respiratory, digestive, and elimination)
- Helps with stress management
- Increases flexibility of muscles and joints
- Increases inner awareness
- Enhances your ability to handle life's difficulties with greater ease
- Enables you to integrate your mind, body, and spirit into one system
- Improves concentration through meditation

There are many Web sites and resources available that can help you understand Kundalini yoga better and prepare you for your first class. Keep an open mind, and allow yourself to experience the benefits and to grow. Experience other forms of yoga as well, because there are many benefits that can be gained by consistent practice. Enjoy your class and keep a journal of your experiences.

PRACTICING KUNDALINI YOGA AT HOME

Even if you don't have any experience with yoga, you can still do meditations and practice the breathing techniques discussed above in the comfort of your own home. You can learn more about the effects these techniques have on your body. Check the Web sites and resources listed at the end of this chapter to explore further.

Those who do have experience with yoga may feel comfortable with creating a yoga set for your own self-care. There are many Kriyas that you can put together to design a yoga program that is specific to your needs. You can change Kriyas every week, every month, every quarter, every year. The changes you make are up to you! Feel free to use the sample class described in this chapter as a guideline.

Morning Sadhana

There is a practice in Kundalini yoga called the morning Sadhana. This is a form of self-care for all Kundalini yoga teachers and students. It allows us to self-heal by working on our physical bodies and also gives us the deep meditative experiences that make us self-aware.

> The process of self-healing is the privilege of every human being. Self-healing is not a miracle, nor is it a question of being able to do something that most people can't. Self-healing is a process that occurs through the relationship between the physical and the infinite power of the soul. It is a contract, a union—that is the science of Kundalini yoga.

Before or around 4:30 in the morning, yoga teachers and students awaken to practice yoga, meditate, chant, and set the pace for their day to begin. Often they take a cold shower for 2 to 5 minutes, before they perform the Sadhana or any yogic exercise. This is called Ishnaan therapy, and this helps to awaken and stimulate the body. The Sadhana is best done during the hours of 3:30 and 6:30 a.m. because it is quiet then and we can draw on the peaceful energy of our Golden Chain. Don't be intimidated by the early morning hours. Sadhana is your own individualized yoga practice and can be done whenever you are able. It is best to discipline yourself by picking a time for your Sadhana and then sticking with that time. It takes a great deal of discipline to get up early in the morning or to perform a daily yoga practice, so the Sadhana serves to help us be disciplined. The Sadhana is preferably performed early in the morning before you start your day, but if you work nights, you can do it a few hours before you would have to get up for work. You should not pick a time for the Sadhana just for the sake of convenience. The main idea is for you to make a sacrifice to do something for yourself that helps improve your health and self-discipline and to set your day up for success. Create your own personal Sadhana with the tools you have been given in this chapter, from books you have read, or from online resources you have found. A Sadhana includes reading, Kriyas, and meditation.

Ishnaan therapy

Even if cold showers don't sound appealing to you, try to be open-minded and experience this activity at least once. You never know—you just might like it! This is another tool that can bring many benefits to your body that you might not have been aware of. It can increase circulation to your vital organs, aid in flushing toxins from your system, and stimulate the flow of purified blood to those organs. You will find that your blood circulation is greatly improved, your lymph system is moving, your nervous system is balancing itself, you are more energetic, and your digestive tract is stimulated.

Ishnaan therapy exercise

1. Wake up in preparation for the morning Sadhana.
2. Take a sponge or brush and exfoliate your skin before getting in the shower.
3. Next, take almond oil and rub it all over your body.
4. The shower should last about 3 minutes to 5 minutes. (Underwear or shorts can be worn to maintain the thighbone magnesium–calcium balance.)
5. Keep your body moving for the duration of the shower using your hands and feet to massage yourself all over (you can also do the Breath of Fire to heat yourself up while you're in the shower).
   (Adapted from "Yogic Lifestyles: The Amazing Cold Shower!" http://www. Spirit Voyage.net)
6. Record your experience in your journal.

Note: Women should avoid taking cold showers when menstruating.

FURTHER STUDIES IN KUNDALINI YOGA

Yogi Bhajan believed that the way to become a better student of yoga was to teach it. He often would say, "If you want to learn something, read it. If you want to understand something, write about it. If you want to master something, teach it." The Kundalini Research Institute (KRI) Level 1 Teacher Training Program is one way to further your knowledge through study and application of daily yogic practices. The class is about 200 hours, which might be subject to change. The class includes 160 hours of direct classroom instruction from a certified Kundalini yoga instructor.

You can do independent study, projects, and practice on your own to complete the required hours. Presenters from other areas and ashrams also come to be a part of the training experience. Classes vary according to the location, teacher, and student circumstances. Usually they are held twice a month for about 7 months, with a few weekends included.

Three books are required for training: *The Aquarian Teacher – Level 1 Yoga Manual, Level 1 Textbook*, and *The Master's Touch*. All of these books were written by Yogi Bhajan and are reviewed thoroughly during the teacher training program. When you complete your yoga training, you receive a full membership in the IKYTA. To find a training program, contact 3HO or visit the Web site to find a class near you. To fulfill the requirements for KRI teacher training, you must:

- Complete class attendance.
- Create your own yoga set that you will practice for 40 days, as well as a personal Sadhana that you will practice for 40 days and record in your journal.
- Complete 20 Kundalini yoga classes outside of your teacher training with other certified Kundalini yoga teachers or at the ashram.
- Participate in a day of White Tantric yoga.
- Be a member of the IKYTA.
- Complete payment for the course.
- Attend five morning Sadhanas at the center where you are studying.
- Pass the KRI examination.
- Complete a confidential evaluation of your teacher/trainer.
- Conform to the Code of Professional Standards for Kundalini yoga teachers.
- Complete a satisfactory practicum assessment.

White Tantric Yoga

One of the major requirements for teacher training is to learn White Tantric yoga. When we think of "tantric," we usually think of ancient sexual practices. However, Tantric yoga is not sexual by any means. The purpose of this yoga practice is to break down any subconscious blocks, behaviors, or patterns that don't suit our needs. When these blocks are released, we are able to be who we truly are and enjoy our lives more completely. We can live every day unaware of the power of our thoughts and sabotage our careers, relationships, and happiness without recognizing it. White Tantric yoga is a series of exercises that help to speed up our progress in healing, which otherwise might take years.

The unique feature of White Tantric yoga is that the participants are arranged in a special formation that allows the energy of each person to strengthen and support the other in the group. White Tantric yoga reminds me a lot of the domino effect. The energy is directed through an individual and begins to move through other individual like a chain reaction. Once a domino falls over, it is done. The difference between White Tantric and dominoes is that instead of tipping over like a domino, each individual remains supported and energized. Yogi Bhajan was called the Mahan Tantric, or Master of White Tantric yoga. He described it as follows:

> Envision the energy of the universe as both parallel and perpendicular in nature, like a cloth woven together. As a cloth becomes stronger when it is stretched on the diagonal, so the White Tantric Yoga® diagonal, or 'Z' energy is stronger. This energy, when directed by the Mahan Tantric, cuts through the blocks that are stuck in the subconscious mind. Using the diagonal energy, the Mahan Tantric, Yogi Bhajan, connects his subtle body to the subtle bodies of the participants through the course facilitator. This works the same way as a worldwide telephone system that relies on satellites and electromagnetic energy in order to connect two parties" (Bhajan, How it works).

White Tantric yoga is done in pairs, with the partners mirroring each other. The combination of partners is not based on the sex of the individuals. This helps activate the diagonal energy of the group. The workshop consists of six to eight Kriyas that are 31 to 60 minutes long. The Kriyas may include all the components in a yoga class that we have discussed already, such as Asanas, Mudras, Pranayamas, and mantras. A trained facilitator serves in proxy for Yogi Bhajan, and a videotape of Yogi Bhajan is played periodically in which he or she gives instructions for each exercise while sharing his or her insights on the experience at hand.

ASSOCIATIONS FOR KUNDALINI YOGA PRACTITIONERS

The following associations may be useful for furthering your studies in Kundalini yoga. There are specific associations and foundations that conduct research and are specific to healthcare professionals. Explore them all and learn more about the Kundalini yoga experience. Don't forget to study other schools of yoga too!

Association for Kundalini Yoga Practitioners
3HO IKYTA
6 Narayan Court
Espanola, NM 87532
Phone: 505-629-1708
Fax: 424-731-8348
E-mail: ikyta@3ho.org

3HO Foundation – Happy, Healthy, Holy Organization
http://www.3ho.org
6 Narayan Court
Española, NM 87532
Phone: 888-346-2420; 505-629-1709
Fax: 424-731-8348
E-mail: YogaInfo@3HO.org

Guru Ram Das Center for Medicine and Humanology (for healthcare professionals)
http://www.grdcenter.org
P.O. Box 1926
Espanola, NM 87532
Phone: 800-326-1322
E-mail: healthnow@grdcenter.org
• http://www.kundaliniyoga.com
• http://www.whitetantricyoga.com

REFERENCES

Bhajan, Y. (1997). *The master's touch: On being a sacred teacher for the new age.* Espanola, NM: Kundalini Research Institute.

Bhajan, Y. (2005). *The Aquarian teacher: KRI international Kundalini yoga teacher training.* Espanola, NM: Kundalini Research Institute.

Bhajan, Y. (2006). *Kundalini yoga for youth and joy.* Espanola, NM: Kundalini Research Institute.

Bhajan, Y. (2007). *Kundalini yoga Sadhana guidelines: Create our daily spiritual practice.* Espanola, NM: Kundalini Research Institute.

Nichols, H. (2008). *White Tantric yoga: A kundalini yoga meditation technique.* Retrieved May 25, 2009, from Suite101.com: http://meditation-techniques.suite101.com/article.cfm/white_tantric_yoga

SUGGESTED READING LIST

Bhajan, Y. (2006). *Kundalini yoga for youth and joy.* Espanola, NM: Kundalini Research Institute.

Bhajan, Y. (2007). *Kundalini yoga sadhana guidelines: Create your daily spiritual practice.* Espanola, NM: Kundalini Research Institute.

CHAPTER 8

Introduction to Herbal Self-Care

RACHEL Y. HILL

"The best medicine you will ever take is the medicine you make."
—KAHLA WHEELER – PRAIRIE WISE HERBAL SCHOOL

MY PERSONAL STORY

I was born in the early seventies and missed the hippie era because I was too busy being a child. I am almost certain, given the way I behave now, that I would fit in with all the groups of nature lovers from that era. Since I took my first herbal class 5 years ago, I have found myself talking to my plants, carrying pictures of them to help establish a closer relationship, and doing little exercises to listen to and honor Mother Earth. Sound crazy? I'll be the first to admit that it is a little crazy, but it is so fun to connect with plants in this way. I once attended a spiritual retreat called Sanctuary of Hope. The high point of my week, and a unique experience for me, was when I hugged a tree. Tree hugging isn't something I ever thought I would do, and I know that I've probably made fun of those "tree-hugging" people I'd read about in the past. Later, an incriminating picture of a group of us hugging a tree happened to show up in my Healing Touch Level 4 class. In the picture, my feet are bare and my face is smashed against the trunk of the tree, almost as if we were meshed as one. I can remember being so close, because I wanted the tree to speak to me and I knew it had an important message to give me. The message I received was unspoken, but it was there. I felt an amazing pull inward, like the tree was welcoming an old friend. What people don't realize is that there is an unspoken magic in Mother Nature's connection with all living beings. If you immerse yourself in nature, she will speak to you through the animals, the wind, the water, the bugs, and especially the herbs.

Herbs have been an important part of my life for as long as I can remember. I have very fond memories of taking hot summer walks with my grandmother Odessa Crith, picking vegetables from the neighborhood garden in Topeka, Kansas. I remember the leathery texture of the deep, green collards she used to pick. I remember the section of corn she kept growing in a tiny patch in her backyard. She'd make a delicious spicy relish called Cha-Cha. Grandmother Crith had a way

185

of making vegetables taste so good, I was eating vegetables that no kid in my school had ever heard of. I loved okra, jalapenos, eggplant, and green tomatoes. I ate them as readily as I would eat an orange or an apple.

I would often watch my grandfather Vaughn as he worked diligently in his garden. I would see him bury fish heads in the soil to fertilize his rose bushes and flowers. I would feel bad because the little beady eyes of the fish would be staring at me from the pits in the soil. Before he covered them with dirt, it appeared to me as if they were looking up at me, asking me to rescue them. I felt bad for the fish, but there was no denying how beautiful his rose bushes were every year.

During the cold and flu season, my mother always kept a purple onion (cut in half) on the windowsill. My grandmother Legusta would keep crabapples in select corners of the room to keep rodents away. Whenever someone had a fever, she would cover him or her with peach leaves. She would also give him or her mullein plant to smoke, just as the Indians used to. Mullein has healing properties and is beneficial for use in respiratory conditions. I always thought of these practices as weird but tolerable. Now I have come to appreciate my grandparents' ways because I realize the value in them. They used nature to the fullest extent for our nourishment, healing, and protection.

HISTORY OF HERBALISM

The history of herbalism goes back about 5000 years and then some. In 2800 BCE, Pen Ts'ao of Shen Nung wrote about 366 different descriptions of plants and their uses. Galen (129–200 BCE), physician to the gladiators and Marcus Aurelius, categorized plants and disease into four humors (hot, moist, cold, and dry) and degrees (first, second, third, and fourth). Paracelsus (1493–1541), doctor, mystic, and surgeon, believed that plants grow in areas where they are needed by others, and that knowledge can be gained not only from books but also from the wisdom of older people and cultures. Nicholas Culpeper (1616–1654 BCE), an apothecary, believed that plants had outer and inner qualities. Some of the more recent teachers of herbalism who have influenced our thinking about herbs are Rosemary Gladstar, Susan Weed, Kahla Wheeler, and many more I have not mentioned (Wheeler, 2001).

Kahla Wheeler, the founder of Prairie Wise Herbal School, has been my herbal teacher for the past 5 years. I have such wonderful memories of a group of us standing in her kitchen, gathering around in a circle to sing "A Farmer's Grace" before our organic potlucks. The aromas of the foods we share blend with one another and saturate the air. Let's just say it makes it very difficult to concentrate in class (that is, until lunch is served). Before we eat, we always join our hands together in a circle and sing "A Farmer's Grace" (or as much as we can remember of it). Kahla belts the old folk tune out like she is giving a concert. The words of the song are as follows:

A Farmer's Grace

The silver rain, the golden sun,
The fields where scarlet poppies run.
And all the ripples of the wheat,
Are in the bread that I do eat.
So when I sit for every meal,
With grateful heart, I always feel,
That I am eating rain and sun,
And scarlet fields where poppies run.

As you can tell, through my lessons from Kahla, I'm learning a great deal about nourishing the body with the help of Mother Nature. Time and work had taken me so far away from the way of life I had observed through my grandparents. Herbs can be used as both food and medicine. What we put in our bodies has a great deal to do with our mental, physical, and spiritual well-being. Unfortunately, with limited knowledge about the properties of herbs, people can be misguided or misinterpret their own information. Adverse reactions and drug interactions can cause people to be very avoidant in exploring herbs to a greater extent. People will sometimes try an herb they have heard about, and think that taking more of it will solve their problems. In most cases, it usually doesn't. The use of herbs is a lifestyle change, not a quick fix. Knowledge is the key, and nurses can be instrumental in integrating herbalism back into the healthcare setting. Pharmaceutical companies, nurses, and physicians should come together and explore safe ways to integrate natural medicine into the regimens of patients. This, however, is a project that will take some time and more research on safe ways to proceed. In the meantime, nurses should take the opportunity to incorporate nature and herbs back into their lifestyle and develop a knowledge base so that they can help people in need of information.

The first lesson I learned from Kahla, in my herbal class, came from the work of Susan Weed (1989). Susan teaches from the perspective of a woman full of wisdom and knowledge. She has a very deep and profound relationship with plants that always speaks through her writings. According to Susan, there are three traditions of healing: the scientific, the heroic, and the wise woman. In the scientific tradition, we trust in machines and what science can do to cure us, and death is considered a failure. Medicines are an important component to this model because they can rid individuals of their symptoms. There is an old saying that evolved from the beginning of the medicine era: "Take two aspirin and call me in the morning." This symbolizes the transition when medicines became more valued than herbs in our society.

THREE TRADITIONS OF HEALING

In this chapter, we will talk about ways that herbs can help bring comfort, relaxation, and nourishment to our bodies. You should always consult with a physician and clinical herbalist before embarking on any type of herbal regimen. The use of herbal supplements can get a little complicated because some herbal supplements are standardized and some are not. You should not even take the standardized herbal supplements unless you are knowledgeable and have been informed about their implications and how they might interact with any medications you are currently taking.

The theme of the heroic tradition is to "save the day" and make someone better. The healing is coming to the rescue. You're sick? Let's give you a special concoction that will make things better. These measures are along the line of poking, puking, and purging to achieve balance. An example of this would be colon cleansing. My grandmother would always want to give us a laxative when we were sick. This was the healing tradition that was common for her time. As in the scientific tradition, death is also seen as a failure because the effort to cure did not work.

In the wise-woman tradition, the wise woman nourishes her family's health through the use of food as the first line of defense. This chapter is not specifically about nutrition, but it is about integrating herbs (which are considered food) into our lives for self-care. Our self-care is based on nourishing the body and helping to restore the balance we need, from a natural perspective. In the wise-woman tradition, we are much larger than the sum of our parts. This is also a common theme in holistic nursing. We are whole beings—body, mind, and spirit. I am in total agreement with the idea that "you are what you eat." We are also what we think, what we surround ourselves with, and so on. Most importantly, what we put into our bodies is seen as a significant factor in our health status. The wise woman does not attempt to cure; she embraces death as a victory and celebration of life. Other traditions consider death a failure. In the wise-woman tradition, curing others is not the priority. The priority is to take in an adequate supply of nutrients into the body and to rely on the body's subtle messages of what it needs from you at that time. You may be feeling water retention in your body, and you drink dandelion for relief. You are not robbing your body of important electrolytes like some diuretics might, when excess fluid is released. In fact, you are putting vitamins, minerals, and nutrients (potassium) into your body. Your body may be telling you to take a day of rest, and a full day of rest helps to prevent you from developing a cold. When you listen to your body and give it what it needs, curing is often a positive and natural side effect. What do the traditions of healing have to do with self-care? I can see a little of myself in each category, but the wise-woman tradition of healing resonates with me. This is what I see so many nurses doing already in their interactions with others. I am sharing this perspective with you, so that you can consider practicing the same wisdom that you share with others. Hippocrates was very intuitive when he said, "Let medicine be your food, and food be your medicine." Herbs are best used as food sources that serve to nourish and tone our bodies, but they can also provide benefits of comfort, relaxation, and healing.

There is so much to know about herbs, further study is advised if you decide to incorporate herbs into your daily regimen of self-care. Here we will discuss the basics of using herbs to make you feel good (legal herbs of course!) and show you how to incorporate a few simple uses safely into your self-care practices. The secret to herbalism is to keep things simple when you first begin to explore herbs. There are so many herbs at our disposal, with so many beneficial properties our bodies can use that we can be tempted to throw them all in one big pot and try to use them all at once. This zealousness can keep us from experiencing the benefits and properties of each herb, so that we know how each one can help us. Using one herb at a time also helps us identify if an herb does not agree with us or causes an allergic reaction. In the herbal community, we call this the "Simpler's Method." We practice keeping things simple by exploring one herb at a time. In my basic herbal classes, I would pick one herb per week and get to know that herb in a special way. I remember my first herb was the sunflower. I ate sunflower seeds for a whole week, used sunflower oil, put sunflower seeds in my salad, kept a sunflower on my kitchen table, and wore a sunflower apron when I cooked. To top it all off, I live in Kansas, where the state flower is the sunflower. How much more connected to a plant could you get?

Common Terms Used in Herbology

Blend – A combination of more than one herb mixed together.

Decoction – An infusion of simmering roots and/or bark boiling in a menstrum of water for 15–30 minutes to draw the nutrients out to nourish the body.

Harvest – Collecting plants and herbs at certain times of the year or season.

Herbology – The study of herbs.

Infusion – A tea or decoction of herb parts that are boiled for an extended period of time to obtain nutrients from them.

Menstrum – The medium used to pull the nutrients from the plants.

Nourish – To fortify the body with nutrients that it needs.

Tea – An infusion of flowers and/or leaves boiled in a menstrum of water for 10–15 minutes, for nutrition or relaxation.

Tincture – An infusion of herbs extracted in a menstrum of alcohol to draw the nutrients out.

Tonic – An herb that tones the body.

What is Herbology?

Herbology is the study of herbs. In herbology, you learn about many parts of a plant that can be used for self-care. The leaves, roots, flowers, and seeds can all contribute to health and well-being when used properly. These different parts of the herb can be used to make different products for use externally or internally. Herbs can be taken in many different ways. They can be made into capsules, pills, lozenges, suppositories, salves, balms, lotions, decoctions, and teas.

Plant Medicines for Relaxation and Healing

Tea

Almost everyone drinks tea at some point in his or her life. Some people like iced tea, brewed in the sun on a hot summer day. Some people like to enjoy a nice quiet teatime with an assortment of tea bags and scones or crumpets on the side. Either way you like to drink your tea, there are a few specifics you probably didn't know. Teas can be broken down into two categories based on the parts of the herb being used: teas (or infusions) and decoctions. Leaves and flowers are used to prepare teas and infusions. Decoctions are made with the roots and bark of the herb, and are usually stronger in flavor. Another difference between the two is that teas are steeped and decoctions are simmered.

Making tea infusions

Tea is an infusion. First, select the herb for your tea infusion. Place the herb in a tea ball, tea strainer, or tea bag (paper or muslin) that will keep the herb and water separated, and put that into a teapot or cup. Bring water to a boil. Pour hot water into the cup or pot, cover, and let the tea steep for about 10–15 minutes. Then simply remove the herbs, sweeten the tea with honey or sweet leaf (optional), and enjoy.

Herbal teas have many benefits. They provide us with nourishment for our bodies, their warmth can be very soothing, and they also provide us with the benefits of relaxation. Because herbs are, in a sense, food, they give the body many vitamins, antioxidants, and nutrients. I have found myself craving certain herbs. I will make teas of them and drink them until my body says "no more."

When this happens, I know that I have probably been mineralized and am full of what I needed from that herb. But as soon as I finish with one herb, I often find myself craving a different one. Teas can serve as tonics that work to tone the body's muscles, organs, and systems. Kahla Wheeler said, "I have found that drinking infusions reduces my desires and cravings for food that are not packed with nutrition" (Wheeler, 2001).

Some examples of single teas to try are chamomile, lavender, peppermint, lemon verbena, lemon grass, lemon balm, ginger root, dandelion, and cinnamon. By trying single teas first, you can better assess your reactions or sensitivities to particular herbs. Before you make any herbal formulation, do your homework and study each herb you have chosen to experience. Figure 8-1 illustrates all the questions you should answer to familiarize yourself with the herb. This can become your own personal material medica, or herbal journal, in which you store all your herbal information, stories about your experiences with an herb, and the effects an herb has had on your life. Every herb you experience can become a part of your herbal record.

Figure 8-1   Materia Medica Sheet

Materia Medica

Plant's common name:
Botanical name:
Family name:

Plant actions:

Part of plants used:
Geographical location and harvesting of the plant:
Medicinal uses or indications:

Preparation:

Special indications or instructions:
Constituents:

Folklore, legend, & science stories:

Personal stories/experiences:

Before we get started with our self-care exercises, we should talk about the ways in which we can capture the nutrients from the herbs. We can and do eat herbs directly, which is a sure way to reap their benefits. We can also use menstrums. The menstrum is the substance in which the herb is soaked so that the nutrients can be extracted. Water and alcohol are the most commonly used menstrums. Tea is made with a water menstrum, and tinctures are made in alcohol. The nutrients of the plant are drawn into the menstrum. The herb is separated from the menstrum, which is then full of nutrients that can be used externally or for consumption. Oil, vinegar, and honey are also good menstrums for extracting the nutrients from herbs for common use.

Self-Care Exercise for Tea

Teatime! We are going to make a simple tea infusion (relaxation/sleepy-time tea). Purchase dried chamomile from your local health-food store or grocery. There are two types of chamomile: German (*Chamomilla recutita*) or Roman (*Chameaemelum nobile*). Chamomile helps to reduce digestive discomfort and improve liver function, and is often consumed after dinner. I always drink it to help me rest at night.

You can purchase chamomile tea bags, but the loose flowers will ensure a better buy. I have opened some tea bags and felt like I needed to look for the herb, because it was so scarce. The dried flowers are bright yellow and white. They smell heavenly to me! (Speaking of heavenly, chamomile has very beneficial effects on allergic rhinitis. So inhale your cup of tea before you drink, and take advantage of the soothing properties it has on the nasal mucosa.) Follow the instructions above for making a tea infusion and be on your way to relaxation. For a single cup of tea, you can add 1 cup of boiling water (Hawkey, 2002) to 1 teaspoon of dried chamomile or 2 teaspoons of fresh chamomile. Have your own individual teatime or share your teatime with your coworkers. Nothing enriches a day like offering to fix some tea for a friend. Create a ritual around teatime at home or at work, and make that a special time for yourself. If you have little girls (or big girls), have a tea party and recapture your inner child. You can go to your sacred space, drink your tea, and listen to relaxing music of your choice. Most importantly, experience the tea, the flavor, the aroma. Listen to what the herb has to say to you, how it makes you feel inside, and how your body seems to respond to it. Write the experience down in your journal!

Decoction

The word decoction comes from the Latin word for "I cook." The simmering time for a decoction takes a little longer, because you are drawing the nutrients out of the roots and bark. "This process is appropriate for harder plant parts, such as twigs, bark, seed, and roots, which require the pressure of sustained heat to coax their chemicals out into the tea" (Crawford, 1997).

Making a decoction

It generally takes 15–30 minutes to make a decoction. Place the dried herbs (roots and/or bark) and water in a pot (avoid aluminum). You can use 1 ounce of dried herb in a pint of water. More water can be added to make sure the herb is covered. Cover the pot and allow the herbs to simmer. Once the herbs have simmered, strain the water into a container. I usually use decoctions when I am not feeling well. I make a big pot and drink the decoction for an entire day. Two to four times a day is what is suggested for drinking a decoction. This is a very nourishing way to incorporate herbs into the diet.

Self-Care Exercise for Decoctions

For this exercise, we are going to make a decoction. Decoctions made from roots can be bitter. I sometimes mix a little honey in with my decoctions, to make them go down nice and smoothly (or as smoothly as possible). You don't have to use the herb I chose for this exercise—you can pick your own root or bark. I chose to use Burdock root (*Arctium lappa*). The plant takes 2 years to complete its life cycle. The first year, it has leaves only, which can be mistaken for rhubarb. The leaf stalks have purplish, reddish veins. There is a white undersurface that is dense and differentiates it from rhubarb (Weed, 1989). The second year, it will flower. Burdock is a nourishing tonic that aids the digestive tract, helps clear the skin, and supports the liver, lungs, kidneys, female reproductive system, and joints. Follow the directions for making decoctions. For burdock root, you can take 1–9 teaspoons (or 5–45 mL) each day.

Other Herbal Exercises for Self-Care

Nature walk—meet your neighbors

Whenever I am feeling really connected and on top of the world, and also when I am feeling stressed, I like to go out in nature and take a walk because it helps me keep things in perspective. It never fails that I am able to see a part of nature that speaks to me and gives me one more thing to be grateful for, and lets me know how magnificent creation is. Next time you feel stressed or just feel like bonding with Mother Nature, take a walk and see how many things you can notice about nature and the plants that are in your surroundings. Look at the ground and try to remember how many plants you saw. Do your best to remember their descriptions. I have a camera on my phone and often find myself taking pictures when I discover plants I have never seen. You can take pictures too. When you finally make it home, look them up. This will be the start of becoming acquainted with your "new neighbors and friends," the plants. Once you have figured out what they are, go back again and reintroduce yourself! Record your experience in your journal.

Tree-hugging exercise

This exercise is as simple as it sounds. Find a tree that looks like it needs a hug and hug it. Spend some time with the tree and listen to what it has to share with you. Forget about what all the people driving by think! Just enjoy the experience.

Herbal bath salts

After a long day at work, your feet may tend to ache and feel a little stiff. This foot soak is simple and excellent for invigorating and comforting the feet. Put ½ cup of Epsom salts and ¼ cup dried lavender into a bag made of cheese-cloth or muslin, or even a sock. You can add a few drops of lavender essential oil to the mixture if you wish. Toss the bag into a nice hot bath and enjoy.

Salad fixin's

Since we now have you drinking teas and decoctions, let's incorporate herbs into your mealtime. There are so many things you can make from herbs that are both tasty and good for you. Experiment by making a salad using dandelion greens, sunflower seeds, lavender, jasmine, or dill, or any herb you like. Enjoy the flavors you experience, and write about how you feel about the new friends you are making in the plant kingdom.

HERBAL CONSULTATION FOR SELF-CARE

Selecting an Herbalist

Another alternative for self-care is to consult with a clinical herbalist. You can find an herbalist the same way you would find any other holistic practitioner—online or through holistic directories. Herbal or health-food stores in your neighborhood may also have listings that can point you in the right direction.

Pricing for Herbal Consultations

Herbal consultations can range from $50 to $250 (and up) and can include a range of other services. Sometimes the herbalist will recommend herbal remedies for you to take after your consultation, so that you can get started on an herbal regimen.

Duration and Frequency of Sessions

Consultations usually last 1–2 hours and may include some follow-up appointments, depending on the arrangement. Some issues can be resolved with weekly sessions. More chronic conditions may require bimonthly or monthly sessions.

Further Studies

I am completing my studies with Kahla Wheeler at Prairie Wise Herbal School (www.prairiewise.com). This school is located in Leavenworth, Kansas. There are many programs that are available to further your information if you desire to learn more about herbs and incorporate them into your life in greater detail. The best source of information is the American Herbalists Guild (www.americanherbalistsguild.com). This is a one-stop shop for finding a study program or herbalist. The American Botanical Council (www.abc.herbalgram.org) has a wealth of information about continuing education opportunities for herbal studies. There are many well-known herbalists, but two names to know are Rosemary Gladstar and Susan Weed, who both offer herbal programs that provide very enriching experiences. Rosemary Gladstar is the director of the Sage Mountain Herbal Retreat Center and Botanical Sanctuary (www.sagemountain.com). Susan Weed is the founder of the Wise Woman Center (www.susanweed.com), which provides information regarding herbal programs in the Wise Woman tradition. I hope that after reading this chapter, you will continue to bond with plants and see them in a different light—after all, you have hugged trees now, so you have to see plants differently!

REFERENCES

Crawford, A. M. (1997). *Herbal remedies for women*. Rocklin, CA: Prima Publishing.

Hawkey, S. (2002). *Herbalism: Using herbs for stress relief and common ailments*. London, UK: Hermes House.

Weed, S. (1989). *Wise woman herbal: Healing wise*. Woodstock, NY: Ash Tree Publishing.

Wheeler, K. (2001). *Prairie Wise Herbal School: Basic herbalism 1 workbook*. Kansas City, MO: Pilot House.

SUGGESTED READING LIST

Fallon, S. (2001). *Nourishing traditions*. Washington, DC: New Trends Publishing.

Libster, M. (2002). *Delmar's integrative herb guide for nurses*. Albany, NY: Delmar Publishing Company.

CHAPTER 9

Aromatherapy for Self-Care

RACHEL Y. HILL

Essential Oils — are wrung –

Essential Oils — are wrung —
The Attar from the Rose
Be not expressed by Suns — alone —
It is the gift of Screws —
The General Rose — decay —
But this — in Lady's Drawer
Make Summer — When the Lady lie
In Ceaseless Rosemary –

—EMILY DICKINSON

MY PERSONAL STORY

When I was studying for my nurse practitioner boards about 2 years ago, I picked up a bottle of essential lemon oil to use as my trademark scent for my study time. I wanted to reward myself with an uplifting fragrance for each chapter I read or study question I answered. I would end up rewarding myself quite frequently because I couldn't resist smelling my lemon oil every single time I began to study. If I found I was having difficulty concentrating on the subject matter at hand, I would put a little oil on a Kleenex and take a whiff. I would also smell it for a pick-me-up when I found myself growing tired. Over 3 months of studying, I developed a fascinating relationship with lemon oil. If I went into a patient's home and smelled lemon Pledge or something with a lemony citrus scent, I would begin to have flashbacks of my board materials. I remembered vaguely that essential oils make excellent study tools because they can stimulate memory recall. That makes sense (or scents), because the smell of a sweet potato pie can take me back to my grandma's house during the holidays. Why wouldn't a lemony fragrance take me back to the endocrine section of my board review? The day of my board exam, I had my packet of Kleenex and essential oil ready. I neatly prepared a few tissues with the essential oil and took one out whenever I felt anxious about a question or had a difficult time with the answer. Guess what? With lots of help from many sources, I passed my exam. I know that the essential oils were uplifting to my brain and helped me to access what I needed for that moment in time. Whenever I smell lemon oil, I still have a flashback of my board exams!

HISTORY OF AROMATHERAPY

The art of aromatherapy has been around for thousands of years. Along with the use of herbs, aromatherapy was one of the first forms of medicine. According to Grace (2000), "[t]he oldest distillation apparatus, which was found in Pakistan, is approximately 5,000 years old." The ancient Egyptians were known for their fragrances, cosmetics, and special blends used for relaxation and mummification of the dead. Cleopatra was famous for her baths and the essential oils she used to allure many men of distinction. The Egyptians had a great influence on the Greeks, who also used aromatherapy and herbs for relaxation and cosmetic purposes. Hypocrites (460–377 BC), the father of medicine, studied and used herbs in his practice. He had a great interest in the way oils interact with the body and encouraged people to take baths infused with oils.

In ancient Rome, Claudius Galen treated many injured gladiators with plant remedies and was appointed the personal physician of Emperor Marcus Aurelius. The Romans developed distillation techniques to extract aromatic floral waters, but not essential oils. Dioscorides wrote a book called *De Materia Medica*, which described more than 500 plants. A great physician of Persia, Ali Hussein Ibn Abdullah Ibn Sina (980–1037 AD; known to Europeans as Avicenna), invented a coiled pipe that allowed the distillation of essential oils, as opposed to the floral waters.

Paracelsus (1494–1541) believed in the use of natural medicine to prevent illness and heal the body. He believed that for every illness, there is a plant meant to heal it. He coined the word "quintessence," which means the healing component of the plant.

The Crusades contributed to the spread of aromatherapy in European countries; however, it was banned in many areas because of religious beliefs. "[I]n the Medieval Era the Catholic Church rejected the aromatherapy remedies, because of their belief that every disease is a punishment sent by God" (http://www.aromatherapypoint.com). Anything that was used to alleviate pain and suffering was taken as an attempt to interfere with the work and judgment of God.

Carol Linnaeus (1707–1778), a professor at a university in Sweden, was very skilled in working with medicinal plants. As a medical physician, he had a deep understanding of how lifestyle plays a part in health and wellness.

The father of aromatherapy is said to be René Gattefossé, a French chemist. He came from a family of perfumists and published a book entitled *Aromatherapy* in 1928 (Grace, 2000). He coined the term "aromatherapy," which is still used to this day.

There have been many contributors to the field of aromatherapy in addition to Gattefossé. Native American, Chinese, and African herbal remedies are very much a part of our society as well. Many of today's medicines can be traced back to those rich cultures and their traditional use of aromatherapy and herbs.

WHAT IS AROMATHERAPY?

Cooksley (2002) defines aromatherapy as the skilled and controlled use of essential oils for physical and emotional health and well-being. Cosmetic, aromatic medicine, and therapeutic aromatherapy make up the three branches of aromatherapy. The cosmetic branch of aromatherapy utilizes substances that have aromatic properties but are not necessarily essential oils. Various synthetic substances are used in the cosmetic industry for application to the skin. Most essential oils must be mixed with a base oil, water, or lotion before they can be used directly on the skin. If you don't know much about essential oils, you should not try to make any type of cosmetic formulation.

Practitioners commonly deal with the aromatic medicine branch of aromatherapy. Here, essential oils are used internally and prescribed by a skilled doctor, aromatherapist, or pharmacist who creates specific formulations for specific problems. Symptoms are treated with essential oils, as medication would be prescribed to a patient.

In therapeutic aromatherapy, essential oils are used in a variety of ways to alleviate aches and pains and chronic illness. Therapeutic aromatherapy is the most common form of aromatherapy used by individuals on a daily basis.

What Are Essential Oils?

Essential oils are the essence of a plant. The oils can come from various parts of the plant. Cooksley (2002) describes them as "tiny droplets contained in glands, glandular hairs, sacs, or veins of different plant parts: leaves, stems, bark, flowers, roots, and fruits." Two common essential oils are obtained from sandalwood and cedar trees. I love to use sandalwood incense when I meditate, and I love the smell of cedar wood cabinets and chests. Rose oil comes from the petals of roses and tends to be one of the more expensive essential oils, because it takes so many rose petals to create a small amount of oil. Essential oil can be extracted from glands on the surface of peppermint leaves. In the eucalyptus plant, however, these oil glands are found inside the leaves. Oranges have essential oils in their rind, leaves, fruit, and flowers. These oils are the most noticeable when you bump up against a plant or walk into a room with flowers. The fragrance has a way of beckoning you to come closer.

CONCEPT OF AROMATHERAPY

Aromatherapy is the use of essential oils from plants to provide relaxation, clarity, and rejuvenation of the body, mind, and spirit. These oils can also help to decrease pain and anxiety, lift the mood, and meet various needs in all areas of our daily lives.

Ways of Entry for Essential Oils

Nose

Essential oils enter the body by two pathways: through the surface of the skin or through the nose. Do you remember scratch-and-sniff stickers? I thought it was magical how the smell of pizza could be captured in a sticker. I remember being a very happy camper, scratching my scratch-and-sniff sticker over and over again. Our olfactory system works 24/7. Let's just quickly review the olfactory system. When we breathe in, we take in odors that attach to our cilia or nasal hairs. The neurons send messages to the olfactory bulb and the message goes directly to the limbic brain. This process allows smells to stimulate memories, sensations, and emotions within us. When I walk into my house and smell my kids experimenting in the kitchen, I can actually tell whether we will need to make alternate dinner plans or not. Smells serve to comfort and protect us by helping us draw from our memories and past experiences. Smells also create opportunities for learning and awareness. When I was in nursing school, my instructors would talk about the fruity smelling breath of patients in diabetic emergencies. I didn't have a clue what they were talking about until I experienced such an emergency and noticed the patient's fruity smelling breath. I have also experienced a house fire, and now the smell of smoke creates a heightened sense of awareness within me that tells me to secure my safety.

Skin

The skin has many pores and hairs on its surface that allow essential oils to be easily absorbed into the body. Essential oils are not like a medication that accumulates in your system. They are excreted in the urine, stool, perspiration, and breath. The essential oil is applied to the skin after it has been mixed with a lotion, base oil, or water. The essential oil goes through the skin pores and hair follicles, taken in by little capillaries, and is then absorbed into the bloodstream. It can then exert therapeutic effects on various body systems until it is excreted from the body.

Methods of Delivery of Essential Oils

Inhalation

Essential oils are delivered in five different ways. The first method of delivery is inhalation. This is commonly used during the cold and flu season, when our heads are congested. An example of inhalation would be to put a few drops of eucalyptus oil into a bowl of hot water. Place the bowl in the bathroom sink. Get a moist bath towel, lean over the bowl of hot water, and cover your head with the moist bath towel. Allow the eucalyptus, steam, and moisture to soothe your nasal passages and clear the congestion. That is just one example of inhalation. Imagine the benefits of being stressed and taking in a few drops of lavender essential oil to help you to relax during your shift or at the end of a day.

Compress

A compress is another way to deliver aromatherapy to the body. Compresses and poultices are good for sprains, bruises, burns, insect bites, and other injuries. For a good compress, put 15–20 ounces of hot water in a jar and add a few drops of rosemary essential oil. Pour some of the mixture into a bowl. Put a clean cloth (cheesecloth, gauze, or some other form of linen) in the water to soak. Wring out the cloth to prevent excessive dripping. Place the cloth over the injured area. The essential oil will be carried into your system, with the heat helping to intensify the action of the oil. Dispose of the cloth when done. If you need another application, pour the remainder of the liquid into your bowl. Heat the mixture up again if necessary.

Massage

Massage is probably most people's favorite way to deliver essential oils into the body. The massage therapist will choose an essential oil that is known to have a certain impact on the body, mix the oil with a base oil, and then use it during the massage. There are different methods of massage and hand motions that help with the absorption and circulation of the essential oils. There is a self-care exercise coming up that will start you on making your own massage oils.

Diffusion

Diffusion is another means of delivering oils into the body. I remember when simmer pots and potpourri were all the rage. I had a hard time dealing with those, because there were a lot of synthetic fragrances being mixed in with the potpourri and being used alone. That is a form of diffusion. There are various high-tech diffusers that can be purchased online, as well as simmer pots and ceramic rings that can be burned on light bulbs. You have to be very cautious and make sure you don't burn your house down for the sake of self-care. A few drops of essential oil in a pan of water on the stove works just fine for a diffuser.

Bath

The bath is another method of delivery for essential oils. I love to take baths! I was intrigued by the old Calgon bath commercials featuring a lady who is completely overwhelmed by all the things going on in her life. She is ironing a shirt, the baby is crying, a pot is boiling over on the stove, the doorbell rings, and she has had it up to here. She yells, "Calgon, take me away!" Instantly, she is in a bathtub in the garden of Eden and doesn't even look like the same person.

I remember thinking, "I've got to get me some of that stuff!" That may be a bit of a fantasy, but nevertheless, the bathtub is a good place to soak in a few essential oils and enjoy a few moments of your own personal paradise. Adding four to six drops of lavender, chamomile, or whatever you are in the mood for can turn your bath experience into a therapeutic adventure.

USES OF ESSENTIAL OILS IN SELF-CARE

We already know that essential oils can be used for relaxation. They also can be used as first aid treatments for cuts, scrapes, and bruises. When I worked in the ICU, I was having very bad muscle spasms in my back. I had twisted a muscle in my back during a code blue. My herbal teacher gave me St. John's wort salve and valerian root salve (stinky stuff) for my muscle aches and spasms. Wow! I didn't worry about how I smelled. I was so relieved that the spasms had decreased and my back began to heal. Use essential oils to help you to relax after work, to help you sleep, and in conjunction with meditation. The possibilities for self-care practices you can create with aromatherapy are endless.

Benefits of Essential Oils in Self-Care

Essential oils are very beneficial to nurses because we work around so many germs. The oils have antimicrobial properties that can help boost our immune systems and help us guard against critters we might easily catch otherwise. Each essential oil has a specific property that can bring comfort, relaxation, clarity, and energy to our bodies. Have an issue? I bet there is an essential oil you can explore and apply to your body in a therapeutic way. Exploring these oils can provide us with allies that we can carry with us and use in times of stress. I can tell you that peppermint oil is a godsend when you're in a long meeting and didn't go to bed early enough the night before. Essential oils support our body in every system and on all levels. More research needs to be done so that we can integrate aromatherapy into our work settings with patients, but in the meantime, we can definitely practice aromatherapy on ourselves.

Before beginning your experience with essential oils, there are a few points to remember. The first point is that essential oils are very concentrated. In other words, "a little dab will do ya!" You don't have to use an entire bottle of essential oil; it takes just a few drops to provide you with the results you want. The second point is that they should always be diluted or mixed with an oil base, shampoo, lotion, salve, water, or cream. They could cause irritation to your skin if you do not. Some oils can be used "neat" or undiluted, like lavender, patchouli, or sandalwood. The last point is to watch the sources of heat you use when enjoying your aromatherapy. You don't want to get too relaxed that you fall asleep on a candle or simmer pot. "Candles, simmer pots, and lightbulb rings can catch fire if not properly attended" (Dodt, 1996).

Self-Care Exercises for Aromatherapy

There are many easy ways to incorporate aromatherapy for self-care into our daily lives. The nice thing is that it doesn't take a great deal of time, just a commitment to "follow your nose." Aromatherapy can be as simple as stopping to smell the roses in a garden or enjoying a lavender-scented candle for relaxation. If you haven't experienced the benefits of aromatherapy before, here is an easy and simple introduction for you.

Exercise 1: Aromatherapy on the Go

What you need: essential oils and tissues

1. Go sniff shopping for essential oils in your local health store or New Age store. You can even shop online for essential oils. Purchase a few of the oils that you are drawn to. If you haven't got a clue, pick a few of the oils from the suggested list provided in this exercise for starters.
2. Once you've purchased your oil, take it home and do some research. Read about the herb's origin, where it is grown, what the herb and essential oil have been used for in the past, what plant family it is from, and any other details that can help you establish a connection with it.
3. Once you have introduced yourself to the oil, put a few drops of it on an unscented tissue. Take a big whiff. What are your thoughts? What are your emotions? How does your body respond to the aroma? What memories come to you from your experience? Do you have any memories associated with this scent? What words come to mind when you think and smell this aroma? Think about it and write the experience down in your journal.
4. You can do the same thing with any other essential oils you have purchased. Smelling coffee beans in between sniffing the essential oils helps clear your nose so that you will be ready for the next experience.

This exercise is intended for you to practice at work, at home, in the car, or anywhere you have the potential to be stressed or just want to experience relaxation. Simply put some drops on a tissue and carry it in your pocket wherever you go. Take it out when you need it. Allow yourself to experience the benefits of relaxation. Keep some oils in your locker or desk at work (and at home) so that you can pick the specific one you need according to what kind of day you are having.

Suggested essential oils for this exercise include lavender, cinnamon, patchouli, orange, lemon, vanilla, peppermint, eucalyptus, and rosemary.

Exercise 2: A Peaceful Place

In this exercise you will create your own aromatherapy blend or combination of essential oils. According to Mojay (1997), when combining essential oils, there are three levels of blending. Level one blends are for the aesthetic or perfume benefits. Level two blends of essential oils are used for medical benefit to bring health and wellness to others. Level three blends are considered psychological and spiritual and help us to restore mental and emotional balance. The following recipe is for an inhalation mixture (Cooksley, 2002) that can be incorporated into your breathing exercises and can also be used in exercise 1. Make sure that you don't have a sensitivity to any of the oils used in the mixture.

Four parts lavender essential oil

Two parts Ylang Ylang essential oil

Two parts sandalwood essential oil

One part lemon essential oil

Mix the oils together and store in an amber or blue glass bottle (the dark bottle keeps the light from breaking the oils down as fast). Shake the bottle gently before each use. You can add a few drops of your blend to a lotion, your bath water, a shampoo, or 5 ml of a base oil (olive oil) for a soothing massage.

Once you have made your blend, you can practice some of the breathing and relaxation techniques you have learned in this book, while experiencing the aroma of the blend. You can also put the mixture on a few cotton balls or Kleenex, place them in a little Ziploc, and carry them with you in your pocket. You have a "peaceful place" in your pocket wherever you go.

Exercise 3: Simple and Easy Massage Oil

This exercise will allow you to create your own massage oil. It is always a luxury when we have someone else to give us a massage, but if there is no one around, we can still provide ourselves with some relief. This simple massage oil is easy to make and doesn't take a lot of time to mix up.

What you need: essential oil, grapeseed oil, wheat germ oil, vitamin E oil, and a large dark bottle (the oils break down more quickly in clear bottles).

two third cup of grapeseed oil

one third cup of wheat germ oil

10 drops of vitamin E oil

6 drops of the oil of your particular fragrance

1. Put all of the ingredients into the bottle.
2. Shake well.
3. Massage the skin in circular patterns over the surface of the skin.

This exercise is intended for you to use at home or at work. If you work a 12-hour shift, you might want to rub your feet sometime around the 8th hour. That would give you a pick-me-up for the home stretch. After a bath, you can apply the oil while you are still partially wet, allowing the oils to soak into your skin. If your hands are too dry and brittle from hand sanitizers, you can get some comfort from a soothing hand massage. The possibilities are endless. Explore with the different oils you have and once you are done, get more oils, and even share the ones you have. Always research the oils that you are using, so that you know what impact they can have on your body. Use one oil at a time, until you are sure that you are not allergic to any of them.

Aromatherapy Consultation for Self-Care

You can also visit an aromatherapist for a self-care adventure. This provides an opportunity for you to have a face-to-face talk with an expert in the field of aromatherapy. You can get helpful advice regarding any health- or stress-related issues you might have.

Selecting an Aromatherapist

To find an aromatherapist, you can contact schools of aromatherapy for a directory of their graduates or look in holistic newspapers or online sources. You can also find a holistic practitioner that incorporates aromatherapy into his or her treatment plan.

Pricing of Sessions

Prices for aromatherapy sessions range from $30 to $250 per hour depending on the service provided, the therapist's experience, and the local cost of living. The average price is probably around $65 to $70 per hour.

Duration and Frequency of Sessions

The duration of a session will most likely be 1 hour to 1.5 hours. A detailed intake and health history will be conducted before you, and the therapist will discuss issues you might have to determine how often sessions are needed. Acute cases require frequent visits on a weekly basis, and chronic problems can usually be handled on a monthly basis.

What to Expect During an Aromatherapy Session

You can expect to be interviewed in detail so that the aromatherapist can learn a little bit about you and your health and wellness status. After that, he or she will pick oils that will be beneficial for your experience (while monitoring for sensitivities). The oils will be massaged into the skin, applied to pressure points, and possibly diffused into the air for your therapeutic benefit. You will discuss self-care and arrange for a follow-up appointment if needed.

Purchasing Essential Oils

Many brands of essential oils are available. I became more interested in essential oils when I began making my own soaps. I did my best to purchase only organic oils, but didn't really know what I was getting. The quality may not always be as good as what you think you are getting. When you are purchasing essential oils, there are a few questions you should ask beforehand. I got the following questions from *Energy Magazine* (Smith, 2008) and have found them to be very helpful:

1. Do you grow and distill your own plants? (If they don't grow and distill their own plants, they may not have control over the ways in which they are grown and distilled, they may not know how the plants are grown and distilled, and they may not have much of an interest in how the plants are grown and distilled.)
2. Do you use fertilizers and pesticides? (These toxins can hurt the plants as well as yourself.)
3. Is every batch of oil tested using gas chromatography? (This is a means by which each compound in a plant can be individually identified.)
4. Does the manufacturer abide by the French standards of essential oil distillation? (The French are the experts in distilling essential oils. You may also want to contact schools of aromatherapy and ask for advice about which oils have the highest quality.)

Further Studies in Aromatherapy

I am not a certified aromatherapist. My aromatherapy classes have been integrated into my herbalist and holistic health studies. Many programs and books are available for nursing professionals who wish to further their knowledge in aromatherapy. The American Holistic Nurses Association (AHNA) has endorsed various programs that have met its specific criteria. The Institute of Integrative Aromatherapy is fully endorsed by the AHNA and approved by the American Nurses Credentialing Center. The Institute offers a certificate program led by founders Valerie Cooksley and Laraine Kyle. The program offers 325 continuing education hours, with a very detailed agenda, and personal mentorship from the founders. The price of programs in aromatherapy range from $250 to $2500.

I am excited about the idea of nurses furthering their studies in aromatherapy and other holistic modalities, because I know they will find a way to integrate them into their patient care. I work with an awesome group of women in a women's clinic, and before they perform a procedure on a woman, they get the lavender essential oil out and begin to set the mood for the procedure room. These woman have no herbal or aromatherapy experience—just think what they could do with clinical certification! The potential for finding ways to comfort ourselves and each other is endless.

REFERENCES

Cooksley, V. (2002). *Aromatherapy: Soothing remedies to restore, rejuvenate, and heal.* New York: Penguin Putnam, Inc.

Dodt, C. (1996). *Essential oils book: Creating personal blends for mind & body.* North Adams, MA: Storey.

Grace, U.-M. (2000). *Aromatherapy for practitioners.* Essex, UK: C.W. Daniel Co. Ltd.

Mojay, G. (1997). *Aromatherapy for healing the spirit.* Rochester, VT: Healing Arts Press.

Smith, L. (2008). How to use essential oils for self-healing. *Energy Magazine,* December/January, 18–19.

SUGGESTED READING LIST

Please see bibliography for this chapter.

CHAPTER 10

Dream Interpretation for Self-Care

Rachel Y. Hill

"Dreams are illustrations. . .from the book your soul is writing about you."
—Marsha Norman

MY PERSONAL STORY

When I was in England for my daughter's graduation, I saw a commercial for Vauxwell cars. It was really very clever, because people were going throughout their day finding themselves in various predicaments. With every challenge that arose, the individuals involved simply corrected the situation with some impossible remedy. It was almost like they were in a dream world where anything is possible. For example, a gentleman was trying to squeeze into his garage and couldn't fit. He pushed his back up against the wall and the garage expanded to make room for him. In another situation, a swimming pool was way too small for a group of children, so an adult began filling it with more water until it grew large enough to suit the needs of everyone involved. The car company's slogan is, "Imagine a world where everything changes effortlessly, make the world adjust to you." The commercial reminded me so much of how the mind works to serve us in many ways. Dreams and hypnosis are tools that are used by the mind to help us to achieve and go beyond our limitations. For dreams, it is as simple as being able to envision and pursue solutions without question. The question is, how do we do this?

About 4 years ago, I woke up from a very disturbing dream. I dreamed an escaped convict had broken into my home. He needed a place to hide and possibly wanted to harm me. He asked me if anyone was in the home with me, and I told him no. I lied to him, because I did not want him to know that my children were also there. If he knew there were more witnesses to his identity, he would try to kill them too. My children were downstairs sleeping, and I had every intention of killing the convict before they awoke. I invited him to the kitchen to get something to eat, because I wanted to be close to my knives to defend myself. I offered to make him a sandwich and got my sharpest knife to cut the tomatoes. During our encounter, the man's face would change to three different faces, all on the same body. Each time I saw him, his face would change or rotate to one of the three faces. My youngest son suddenly came upstairs into the kitchen, rubbing his eyes from sleep. He asked me for some water. The convict was startled. I was terrified because I knew he would feel betrayed and be angry with me for lying to him. At that moment, I had to protect my family. While the convict was distracted, I ran toward him with my knife. That is how the dream ended. I woke up in a cold sweat.

Shaken, I got up to get a drink of water. As I walked to the kitchen, I found my front door wide open. It was 4:30 in the morning and I was unable to sleep after that. About 7:00 that same morning, I called a close friend of mine and shared my dream and also told him about my front door being open. He told me that three convicts had escaped from a prison in my area. The convicts were found that morning (between 5:00 and 6:00 a.m.) at a local restaurant less than 5 minutes away from my home. The opened door initially added to my unrest, but later led to my relief. I never went back to sleep that day. My children and I were safe, and I believe I had been protected by something greater than I could imagine. I have not dreamed that way since, but I have never stopped reflecting on the impact that dream had on my life. I will always use my dreams as a reason to stop and examine my life and my thoughts and to evaluate my life's path very seriously.

For as long as mankind has been able to communicate verbally and in writing, we have had evidence of the mystery and sacredness of the dream world. Some of the greatest works in history have come from our nighttime slumber. History shows us that some of the most complex projects ever taken on have been achieved through the act of dreaming and the application of that information. Elias Howe had a nightmare that led to the production of the sewing machine. He had worked on a sewing machine for years, without the satisfaction of completing it. In his dream, a group of savages captured him and threatened to take his life if did not finish the machine. In great fear, he stared at the heads of their spears and noticed they contained eye-shaped holes near the points. When he woke up, he realized that he could pass the thread through the needle close to the point (as opposed to the other end, as in conventional needles), and he also remembered the up-and-down movement of the spears. At last he was able to complete his invention.

Friedrich Kekule von Stradonitz, a German chemist, struggled to figure out the structure of benzene. He dozed off one evening and envisioned the atoms forming long chains that were twisting and turning like snakes, with a snake taking hold of its own tail. He realized that benzene was a closed structure. He had also derived his theory of chemical structures from another dream he had experienced 7 years prior (Moss, 2009). Nobel Prize winner Otto Loewi suspected for years that nerve impulses were controlled chemically, not electrically, and one night he had a dream that led to the creation of design that finally allowed him to test his theory. The idea for the theory of relativity came to Albert Einstein while he was in the simple act of dozing.

There have also been many references to dreams in literature. Stories in the Bible about Daniel and the Lion's Den, Jacob's Ladder, and Joseph and the Coat of Many Colors, as well as *Dr. Jekyll and Mr. Hyde*, *Frankenstein*, and many of Shakespeare's works were all spawned from the dream state. Our music is saturated with references to dreams that allow us to drift into fantasy and connect with the thoughts of our romantic love interest. Remember the Everly Brothers' song "All I have to do is dream. Dream, dream, dream, dream, dream, dream..."? A number of movies have reflected the beauty of dreams, such as "The Wizard of Oz" and "Alice in Wonderland." There are also movies that terrify us so much that we don't even want to shut our eyes at night, such as "A Nightmare on Elm Street," where Freddy Krueger harms people through their dreams.

I think that everyone would agree that dreams play an important part in every human being's life, whether we acknowledge them as a miracle or dismiss them like the air we breathe. The truth remains that we dream, and we dream for a reason. We may think that we don't dream, or are unable to remember our dreams, but that doesn't mean that we haven't actually dreamed, or that someone hasn't had a dream about us. The deal with dreams is simply this: Even though most people dream, we feel no true motivation to take our dreams seriously. However, if we have a nightmare or dream something very startling, we may pay attention and take some sort of action. The emotional attachment to a frightening dream lingers in our memory, whereas a dream about taking a boat on the river may not leave as much of an impression.

Despite the themes in our dreams, many people have a tendency to dismiss them as "matter of fact" happenings. We totally ignore the messages and don't make any correlation with what is going on in our lives. If the dream gives us an obvious message or foretells a future event, we place the dream in a closet of "coincidences," and what do we do with coincidences? We usually convince ourselves to dismiss them and forget about the significance of what has occurred.

HISTORY OF DREAMING

Egyptians had many ancient writings that were utilized to interpret dreams. Special priests were dedicated to interpreting dreams for health and divination purposes. The Egyptians and Greeks both had sleep temples where dreams were sought from the gods for guidance. Individuals would refrain from any substances that would prevent the natural dream from coming through. They would also eat certain foods to induce dream states. Hypnos was known as the god of sleep, and his son Morpheus was known as the ruler of dreams. Hippocrates used dreams to diagnose his patients and knew that they were a link to what was going on with his patients. Artemidorus took this insight a little further and desired to know more about each individual in relation to his or her dreams. He was interested in correlating the personal details of the dreamers with their dreams and the meanings of those dreams. The Romans also had deities that were associated with dreaming. Faunna and her brother/husband, Faunnus, were said to rule the dream world. However, once the Romans accepted Christianity, people were no longer permitted to worship such deities. Of course, there are many stories of how dreams have impacted some of the most influential biblical characters in Christian history.

I first realized the importance of dreams when I was a little girl, studying in my Sunday school at church. We would study various lessons about the dreams and visions that different biblical characters had. I would often think about how amazing these stories were and wonder if my life could change as theirs did through dreaming. My favorite story in the Bible is about a young man named Joseph (Genesis 37:2–4). The story of Joseph takes place around 1562–1452 BCE. Joseph had 11 brothers, but he was his father's favorite. His mother died giving birth to his younger brother. To express his love for his son, Joseph's father gave him a multicolored coat. His brothers were very jealous of this and also disliked Joseph because he would often tell his father when they were not behaving as they should. Of course, no one likes a tattletale, so Joseph was never able to fit into his brothers' circle. Joseph was a dreamer and paid a great deal of attention to his dreams. He had a series of two dreams. In the first dream, he and his 11 brothers were represented by sheaves of wheat. During the dream, their sheaves all bowed down before his. In the second dream, the sun, moon, and 11 stars were all bowing before him. Jacob's interpretation of this dream was that these celestial bodies represented him, his mother, and his 11 brothers. The dreams indicated that one day his brothers were to acknowledge Joseph and be subject to his authority. This didn't make any of his brothers happy, so they conspired to dispose of him in some way. They took his coat, covered it with blood, and deceived the father into thinking Joseph had been killed. They put Joseph in a dark well and eventually sold him into slavery to the Egyptians.

When Joseph arrived in Egypt, he was purchased by a man named Potiphar. Potiphar was the captain of the pharaoh's guard. Joseph became successful very quickly and rose to a position of trust in the household. However, Potiphar's wife had Joseph thrown into jail on false charges, because he refused her sexual advances. While in prison, he was able to rise to a position of favor and was given the job of overseeing the overall operations of the entire prison. He was also the overseer of the pharaoh's butler and baker. One night, both the butler and the baker had strange dreams. Having the gift of dream interpretation, Joseph interpreted their dreams. He said that in 3 days time, the butler would be recalled to his former position, but the baker would be killed. Sure enough, 3 days later, the pharaoh restored the butler to his job and killed the baker. Joseph asked the butler to mention his name to the pharaoh in the hope that he would be freed, but the butler forgot about Joseph.

About 2 years later, the pharaoh began to have very disturbing dreams and could find no one to tell him what they meant. The butler remembered Joseph and told the pharaoh about him. Joseph interpreted the pharaoh's dream as predicting 7 years of good harvests followed by 7 years of famine. The famine would be so severe that it would wipe out all the gains of the good years and then some. The pharaoh trusted Joseph and appointed him to create a strategic plan that would save the people from the terrible famine. Joseph became the second in authority in Egypt, reporting only to the pharaoh. During the 7 good years, Joseph married the daughter of an Egyptian priest. By successfully implementing his strategy when the famine came, Joseph prevented the demise of many people and created the opportunity for the pharaoh to take possession of all of Egypt and its wealth in the process.

The finale of my favorite story takes place when the famine reaches the land of Canaan. Jacob sends his sons (who sold Joseph) to Egypt to purchase food. They did not realize they were buying food from their brother. Joseph put the brothers through various ordeals, such as accusing them of being spies, locking them up for 3 days, and keeping one of the brothers while they go and get their father and Joseph's younger brother. All of these events led the brothers to outwardly discuss their guilt about what they had done to their brother, and their fears that God was punishing them. Joseph overheard them and knew that they entirely at his mercy and that his true identity could soon be revealed to them. Joseph and his long-lost family were reunited and given the best land in Egypt as their home. Thus, Joseph's dreams came to fruition over time. Jacob and his wives, and the 11 brothers and their wives and all their children bowed down before Joseph, who had saved them all and brought them into a land of plenty where they enjoyed generations of peace, prosperity, and abundance.

Some of the greatest accomplishments in history have come from the recall we have of our dreams. "In sleep we have the power, in a perfectly normal way, to get valuable instruction and insight"(Hamilton-Parker, 2000). In the late 1800s, Madame C.J. Walker, an AfricanAmerican woman, was having difficulty with her hair falling out. She had tried many medications, herbs, and ointments in attempt to solve her problem. One night she dreamed that a black man came to her and told her about a mixture of ingredients that would help her hair to grow back. She sent for some of the herbs from Africa and gathered the rest of the ingredients locally. She mixed everything together and began to use it on her scalp. She said that her hair grew faster than she could use it. From this creation, she launched a million dollar industry, helped women to become entrepreneurs, and was able to give a great deal to her community. The School of Metaphysics has produced a film called "The 10 Powers of Dreaming," which reflects on 10 categories of dreamers who have impacted history. The first category is the writer or scribe. Mary Shelley wrote *Frankenstein* in 1816, in response to a challenge by Lord Byron to create a horror story that would scare everyone who read it. This classic was born from a dream Mary Shelley had after accepting Lord Byron's challenge. Another category is the prophet. The movie describes a dream Abraham Lincoln had that foretold his own assassination in a dream, only a few weeks before it actually occurred.

CONCEPT OF DREAMING

I have always considered myself a "bootleg" dream interpreter. When I began to interpret dreams for myself, I first learned from the School of Metaphysics. There are many schools of thought and many theories that shed light on the mystery of dreaming, and these are all very informative and profound. However, I tend to use the method I learned at the school most frequently because it is very simple and has a commonsense approach that resonates with me. In my first lesson, I learned three important things about understanding dreams: First, every dream is about the dreamer. Second, dreams that occur during the night are a reflection of the previous day. Third, everyone dreams, even though they may not be able to recall their dreams, and with persistence, everyone can develop the ability to recall their dreams. This might be quite a bit to swallow, but hopefully things will become clearer for you later on.

What Are Dreams?

What are dreams? Dreams are messages from our inner (subconscious) mind to our outer (conscious) mind. Dreams are a means by which our subconscious mind takes our everyday experiences and speaks to us. It speaks by using symbols for people, places, and things to give us messages that can help us understand what we need to do or change, how to relate to others, and so much more. We sleep for the sole purpose of rejuvenating and allowing our bodies to heal, while our dreams come to help bring awareness to our waking day. Our bodies will work toward healing first. Once the rejuvenation has taken place, the dreams can occur. There are many things that can impact our sleep and prevent us from having a healthy dream state. When we travel from one place to another, our circadian rhythm or internal time clock can be thrown off, and our body can't tell whether it is going or coming. A good remedy for jet lag is simply to take your shoes off and connect with the earth where you are at the moment. Environmentally, we can cause damage to our mental and physical bodies by using drugs, drinking alcohol, and not getting enough rest. Some people have a tendency to "fight sleep," as my mother would say, and always try to do things nonstop.

Benefits of Studying Dreams:

- Self-awareness
- Bringing the spiritual and physical worlds together
- Creating harmony in your external life
- Overcoming challenges and obstacles
- Monitoring your thoughts and consciousness
- Identifying your strengths, fears, weaknesses, etc.

When we have nightmares, it is because we have some issues we need to address in our waking state or day-to-day activities. We remember our nightmares because they are linked to emotions. We always seem to remember the scary details of things, because they are attached to fear. Anything we dream that is just ordinary and matter of fact, we will forget. To cultivate a healthy dream life, self-care is of the utmost importance. The quality of your dreams should be very interesting because of your ongoing self-care activities. The activities and choices you are making are leading you to a harmonious life. If you are not taking care of yourself, the dreams you have will be reflected in the form of cars being out of control, tornados, and different types of animals.

Sometimes people have dreams in which they feel like a dark force is holding them captive and they are unable to break free. They feel paralyzed and unable to move, which can be very frightening. This is a simple phenomenon that occurs when you try to wake up during a sleep cycle. Your body has not yet received the message that you are awake, so it is unable to move and stir to meet the day.

Dream Theorists

It is important to mention three influential dream theorists here. Sigmund Freud believed that dreams were the path to the unconscious. He began to analyze dreams to understand the personalities of individuals as they related to certain pathologies. Carl Jung believed that dreams could help people heal through archetypal symbols that represent different characters. Dreams give us mental images from areas in our life we have repressed for some reason, so that we can deal with them. Gestalt therapy was developed by Frederick Perls. In this form of therapy, you act out the different parts of your dreams. For example, if you dreamed about a car, you act out the role of the car. This allows you to recapture parts of yourself that you had put away. The works of these three men are good resources for furthering exploring dreams.

Terms Related to Dreams

Aspect – A characteristic, quality, or virtue we use to judge ourselves or others.

Conscious mind: – Intelligence as it expresses in the physical level of consciousness. This is the part of the conscious mind that is capable of self-awareness (Condron, 1997).

Dream – A communication from the subconscious mind to the waking mind that occurs during sleep and concerns the conscious state of awareness. This communication is needed to ensure the mental, emotional, and physical well-being of the dreamer (Condron, 1997).

Non-REM sleep – Stages 1–4 of the sleep cycle, before REM sleep kicks into gear. The stages last about 5–15 minutes.

REM – This stage usually occurs about an hour after you go to sleep. Dreams occur during this stage of sleep. REM stands for rapid eye movement, a physical characteristic of this stage of sleep.

Subconscious mind – Intelligence expressed in the inner levels of consciousness, collectively known as the soul. The function of the subconscious mind is to recreate the conscious mind's imaged desires, thus furthering experiences for learning. Its purpose is to permanently store understandings gleaned from conscious experiences (Condron, 1997).

Types of Dreams

We have many types of dreams at different points in our sleeping state. Here are a few examples of common dream categories (http://www.dreammoods.com):

- Daydreams: A level of consciousness that teeters between sleep and wakefulness.
- Lucid dreams: Dreams that occur where you know that you are only dreaming.
- Nightmares: Dreams that indicate a loss of control during the conscious waking period or day.
- Recurring dreams: Dreams that happen over and over to convey a message or reveal a lesson that has not yet been learned.
- Healing dreams: Dreams that are comforting or lead one to keys that can promote balance and wellness.
- Prophetic dreams: Dreams that project an event that will take place in the future.
- Epic dreams: Dreams that are so long and memorable, they are like a screenplay that you remember for many, many years.

Common Themes in Dreams

- Animals: Ways of thinking or being (habits)
- Car accidents: Allowing things in your physical life to control you
- Nakedness: Expressive and honest
- Having sex: Creation
- Dying: Experiencing change
- Giving birth: Manifesting a new idea
- Murdering or being murdered: Causing change to happen without any concept of the end result or consequences
- Teeth falling out: Teeth are the tools we use for eating food and helping us to digest the information we are ingesting; food is knowledge; teeth are tools for digesting information
- School: Schools are places we go to learn things
- Eating: Food is knowledge or information

DREAM INTERPRETATION FOR SELF-CARE

How to Interpret Dreams for Self-Care

Dream Recall

The first key to interpreting dreams is to remember your dreams. Everyone dreams, but it just may take a little practice to bring you up to speed with your dream recall. How do you even begin to remember your dreams, when you can't remember the last time you had one? You will want to begin your journey by keeping a dream journal.

- Get yourself a notebook.
- Use a steno pad that already has a line down the center or purchase a pad and draw a line down the middle yourself. Record the dream on the right-hand side and record the symbols on the left-hand side.
- Each night you will date your journal entry, with the anticipation of recalling a dream.
- Get a dreamer's dictionary to use until the symbols become more familiar to you.

Here are some tips to help you to begin remembering your dreams by getting your subconscious mind involved:

- Set the intention to remember your dreams. Your subconscious mind needs to realize that this is something you plan to do.

- Verbalize your intentions outwardly. Affirmation is another way to begin bringing your subconscious and conscious minds together to accomplish the goal of recalling dreams.
- Make a self-hypnosis tape. A self-hypnosis tape is another tool that works with your subconscious mind to plant suggestions so that you begin to recall your dreams with the support of your subsconscious mind.
- Write a dream affirmation down. When you write things down, you are engaging different parts of your brain. Writing always seems to seal the deal for me. Once you begin to write things down, you put what you want out into the universe.
- Reinforce to yourself the benefits that you will achieve from remembering your dreams.
- Go to sleep relaxed. It can be hard to remember your dreams when your body is tense. Doing progressive relaxation exercises will help with relaxation and dream recall.
- Wake to remember your dreams and record them. When you wake up in the morning, rise from bed slowly and write down your dreams. Getting up too fast can cause you to lose your dream very quickly. If you have a dream and wake up during the night, you will have your journal next to your bed so that you can record the dream any time during the night. Even if you can't recall your dreams immediately, date your journal for the next night, with the anticipation of remembering your dreams.

Recording and Interpreting Your Dreams

There are a few helpful tips that I learned from the School of Metaphysics and a Dream Workshop I attended. Your subconscious mind sends a message to your conscious mind through dreams. When you record your dreams, your conscious mind is receiving what the subconscious mind has to say. As you are recording the dream, get the details fresh off the press (your thoughts). Don't wait until later, because the dream gets convoluted and further away from the truth. Begin to identify the symbols in your dream. I purchased a symbols dictionary to help me initially. Some schools of thought discourage that and advise you to go with your impression of what a dream means to you. I think you should do both. There is no right or wrong way, so follow your intuition. When I record dreams in my journal, I draw a line down the middle of the page. I like to write the dream on the left side of the page and the symbols that I will define on the left-hand side of the page. I will first highlight the symbols within my dream on the right-hand side with a colored highlighter, then I will write that same symbol on the left-hand side of the paper, and finally I will define the symbol on the left-hand side of the paper. The next step is to determine the dream theme, from the feeling of the dream and the overall content of what I have received from the definitions of the symbols. Once you have completed these steps, ask yourself why you are having this dream at this particular time in your life. Sit with what you have received and allow the interpretation of the dream to surface for you. Write a summary of your interpretation on your dream journal entry.

Sample Dreams and Interpretations

Below are a few descriptions of dreams collected from some of my nursing colleagues. Each dream was interpreted by Dr. Terry Martin (School of Metaphysics Faculty, Windyville, MO).

Dream 1

Family nurse practitioner and midwife

I had a dream that I was out of town—I think in North Carolina in the Smoky Mountains area. I was with my friends from nursing school and we decided to go get some food. Since we were from out of town and didn't know anyone in the area, I decided to go topless with only my undies on. Why not, right? Anyway, we get to the restaurant and I know everyone who is working there and I am mortified. (I have never had a naked dream before, so this was really weird!)

Dream 1—Interpretation

This dream indicates the experience of expressing nurturing openly and honestly with freedom. Then there are some attitudes of concern because of what others might have thought about this expression. It would be kind of like someone who has been very open in sharing with someone and then feels a bit strange or uncomfortable about the experience.

Dream 2

Family nurse practitioner

I was somewhere with my best friend, having to say goodbye to her for some reason. We were both crying (myself more), and she was trying to comfort me. We were in a strange location that kept changing—it started in a multilevel parking garage and then progressed to a neighborhood of quadplexes. We were just walking and talking. We never did say goodbye or part—I woke up first. (I have said goodbye to her before when I moved to Colorado for 3 years, and we are not getting back to the same level of friendship, but she used to be my nurse when I was working as an NP.)

Dream 2—Interpretation

This dream has to do with a feeling (due to the experience of emotion in the dream) of separation from a part of the self that is known and very close (best friend).

She describes the scenes as being "strange," which indicates a state of mind that is different from what she is used to. This might be a situation that is new, that she is uncertain about where she will go, how it will impact her future, and seemingly it has the potential for the loss of a part of herself.

Dream 3

Women's health nurse practitioner

I had a dream I was hanging out with Lindsay Lohan and we were going to go out together. We were getting on a bus and she had a lot of liquor, and I commented on the amount of liquor she had. We then ended up at a restaurant where we were to meet my brother and sister, and we were so late that when we got there, they were done eating and we were just hanging out in the lobby wondering what we were going to do next.

Dream 3—Interpretation

This dreamer is part of an organization and needs to give herself a direction. Goals would be important for her and learning to make productive choices that will lead her step by step toward their accomplishment. Having goals would provide this dreamer with the means to actually learn (eat the food) and do something rather than just "hang out."

Dream 4

Family nurse practitioner (yours truly)

Paragraph 1

My girlfriend's uncle passed away, and family members and I were attempting to get to Colorado for the funeral. My mother and other relatives were going, but they weren't taking things as seriously as I would have liked them to. They were going to wait and go the next day, but I was going to drive that night just to be there. My friend's mother called to see if we were going and told me we had 4 hours to leave.

Paragraph 2

I then found myself in a yoga class with a lot of women. My teacher was helping me to do some crunches that I was having a hard time with. She offered some videotapes to help me practice and develop my skills. There was a guy from my old high school behind me doing yoga. He was watching how flexible I was. His name was Harvey. The teacher was reprimanding someone, encouraging her to try harder.

Paragraph 3

I was preparing to go back to the funeral, but only after I finished my class in high school. I was picking out outfits and hadn't made it home from school yet. I found a pretty black and white dress that I dressed up with a white sweater. I was trying to pack a little more, instead of trying to cram it all in at the end. I was also debating about the safety of taking the trip alone versus with others.

Paragraph 4

There was a situation in which I was finally with my friend (the one whose uncle passed) and she had a daughter, a little girl, with a very raspy voice. I told everyone that she was going to be a singer, because her voice was so unique. My friend was trying to save her house from foreclosure. We were trying to come up with truthful excuses to prevent the foreclosure, including the fact that her uncle had passed away. Nothing worked, because we wanted to be honest and there was no good reason to justify her failure to make the mortgage payments.

Paragraph 5

I ended back up with the personal trainer/yoga instructor, who attempted to come up with various ideas to help my friend, and we just sat around thinking that something would break through for her eventually. We vowed to stay there and not leave until we were able to come up with a solution.

Paragraph 6

I then ended up in a kitchen with a chef, cooking gourmet sausages. I don't eat beef or pork, but those sausages looked so good that I would have eaten them anyway. My daughter had made chili that day, so I decided I would fix one of those sausages and eat it with the good chili she had fixed for me. I knew it would not make me sick, even though it was beef or pork, if I did not believe that it would.

Dream 4—Interpretation

Paragraph 1

My girlfriend's uncle passed away and family members and I were attempting to get to Colorado for the funeral. My mother and other relatives were going, but they weren't taking things as seriously as I would have liked them to. They were going to wait and go the next day, but I was going to drive that night just to be there. My friend's mother called to see if we were going, and told me we had 4 hours to leave.

A change has been made and the dreamer has continued to place her attention on what was, so some stagnation has occurred (the funeral). The number 4 indicates stability, so the attention is being brought to the need, which is to become grounded.

Paragraph 2

I then found myself in a yoga class with a lot of women. My teacher was helping me do some crunches that I was having a hard time with. She offered some videotapes to help me practice and develop my skills. There was a guy from my old high school behind me doing yoga. He was watching how flexible I was. His name was Harvey. The teacher was reprimanding someone, encouraging her to try harder.

Conscious aspects of self are gathered in an effort to learn how to build strength of the mind, exercising the mind, which will lead to greater life force being available for the dreamer.

Paragraph 3

I was preparing to go back to the funeral, but only after I finished my class in high school. I was picking out outfits and hadn't made it home from school yet. I found a pretty black and white dress that I dressed up with a white sweater. I was trying to pack a little more, instead of trying to cram it all in at the end. I was also debating about the safety of taking the trip alone versus with others.

The attention has moved back to a point of stagnation, with attention being given to outer expression.

Paragraph 4

There was a situation in which I was finally with my friend (the one whose uncle passed) and she had a daughter, a little girl, with a very raspy voice. I told everyone she was going to be a singer, because her voice was so unique. My friend was trying to save her house from foreclosure. We were trying to come up with truthful excuses to prevent the foreclosure, including the fact that her uncle had passed away. Nothing worked, because we wanted to be honest and there was no good reason her failure to make the mortgage payments.

The little girl represents the idea of becoming more harmonious, and an attempt is being made to retain a particular state of mind.

Paragraph 5

I ended back up with the personal trainer/yoga instructor, who attempted to come up with various ideas to help my friend, and we just sat around thinking that something would break through for her eventually. We vowed to stay there and not leave until we were able to come up with a solution.

The dreamer has come back to the point of learning how to have more life force.

Paragraph 6

I then ended up in a kitchen with a chef, cooking gourmet sausages. I don't eat beef or pork, but those sausages looked so good that I would have eaten them anyway. My daughter had made chili that day, so I decided I would fix one of those sausages and eat it with the good chili she had fixed for me. I knew it would not make me sick, even though it was beef or pork, if I did not believe that it would.

There is knowledge available and the dreamer is receiving it.

Overall, I see a movement back and forth between letting go of the past and moving forward. It seems as though you have challenged the self in a way that has required a lot of energy. Your mind is strong in that you are trying to find a way to draw additional resources to yourself, to learn how to use your mind in different ways. The movement of your attention could very well be the old Rachel who hadn't finished her book to the new Rachel and the energy that is required and needed in the present time period to manifest the finalized book. It reminds me of the last few pushes to bring forth a child. Then there is joy and exhilaration for the new mom!

CONSULTING WITH A DREAMOLOGIST FOR SELF-CARE

The School of Metaphysics conducts ongoing research on dreams, and many of the staff members are skilled in the art of dream interpretation. They operate a National Dream Hotline once a year and also have a Web site (http://www.dreamschool.org) where you can post your dreams and consult with someone regarding their meaning. I encourage you to explore this option and get some support in beginning to explore your dreams. It is fun, and you will find that you will learn so much in such a short time that people will be coming to you to interpret their dreams (especially your patients!). There are also other groups that help others find insight to their dreams. Many Jungian groups can be found online in holistic directories and other listings.

FURTHER STUDIES IN DREAM INTERPRETATION

The School of Metaphysics has a Dreamologist program that provides certification upon completion, enabling one to become proficient in the art of dream interpretation. The program consists of seven courses of self-paced lessons, a series of conference calls, assignments that are completed on the honor system, and the attendance of a special focus session called the "Genius Code Spiritual Focus Weekend." The courses can be completed at your own pace. During the program, you correspond with faculty, become a member of an interactive Web site called "www.Dreamschool.org," and read books assigned by the instructors. The Web site is a helpful resource even if you do not desire to participate in the program. It provides access to message boards and dreams that will sharpen your awareness and open your understanding toward interpreting your own dreams.

REFERENCES

Condron, B. (1997). *The dreamer's dictionary*. Windyville, MO: School of Metaphysics Publishing.

Hamilton-Parker, C. (2000). *Unlock your secret dreams*. New York: Sterling Publishing Company.

Moss, R. (2009). *The secret history of dreaming*. Novato, CA: New World Library.

SUGGESTED READING LIST

Hamilton-Parker, C. (2000). *Unlock your secret dreams*. New York: Sterling Publishing Company.

Morris, J. (2002). *The dream workbook*. New York: Little, Brown and Company.

CHAPTER 11

Holistic Coaching for Self-Care

RACHEL Y. HILL

"You cannot teach a person anything. You can only help him to find it within himself."

—GALILEO

MY PERSONAL EXPERIENCE

There are many people out there who are "closet coaches." These wonderful people have a natural way of coaching others, and can sometimes coach without ever knowing it. Teachers, parents, grandparents, uncles and aunts, and role models in the community often make lasting impressions on the lives of many people. So many people can share the story of how one person made a difference in their life. I remember watching an interview with an actor named Yaphet Koto, who played a cop in a detective/crime show. He said that in his youth, he was heading straight down a path to crime and eventually jail. One day he happened to meet Malcolm X, who told him that he was one beautiful black man. He experienced a shift in his focus, began to pursue acting, and ended his life of crime.

Some people have the gift to inspire you to do just about anything through simple words of encouragement. Their smile, right before you hit the finish line, gives you the needed strength to continue the race. Their firm pats on the back serve as fuel for the journey because they don't push you to try to make it—they make you feel as if you already have.

I will never forget my first-grade teacher, Mrs. Wetchensky. She made me feel like Maya Angelou when I wrote my very first poem for show and tell: "If I were a tree, I could stand and see, all the world around me." She stood up and gave me a standing ovation, and my class followed suit. They clapped for me for what seemed like forever, and then I was given bubble gum for a job well done. That was the springboard for many writing projects and always gives me a warm feeling inside. Words of encouragement from my sixth-grade teacher, Mrs. Lee, helped me get to second place in a spelling bee I initially didn't have the confidence to participate in.

In my freshman year of college, I was terrified of chemistry. The instructor seemed very intimidating to me and difficult to understand. My lab instructor (whom I initially thought might be scarier than my chemistry teacher because she was tiny, red-haired, and moved at the speed of light all the time) showed me a very nurturing side of herself that I truly needed, being a freshman and away from home. She rescued me from my self-defeating fear of failing before she even began to tutor me in chemistry. Once my thoughts shifted, she was able to show me how easy chemistry was, as opposed to how hard I was making it.

HISTORY OF COACHING

In the past 15 years, coaching has been utilized mainly to help people succeed in their careers and/or become effective leaders in business. According to Bark (2008), references to coaching can be found as early as the 1930s. Articles were published that related directly to management training. It makes total sense that businesses would utilize coaching. Training leaders to lead and manage effectively is a vital part of having a strong business. In the 1980s, coaching became more recognized for its use in leadership programs. These programs were intended to improve performance. From the 1990s to the present, the field of coaching has grown more than ever. Individuals want to be successful in their careers and personal lives, and businesses want their employees to be productive for the good of the company. Companies want their employees to tap into their hidden potential.

Coaching isn't just good for businesses—it has branched into many different fields. Here is a list of just some of those area:

- Spirituality
- Weight management
- Health and wellness
- Holistic life coaching
- Life coaching
- Grief coaching
- Parent coaching
- Business/career coaching
- Entrepreneur coaching
- Relationship coaching
- Self-care coaching
- Sports coaching

The fact that the list of different types of coaching keeps growing leads me to believe that people aren't satisfied with being mediocre anymore. It also shows that for every need, there is a coach willing to support others on their journey. People are searching for greater meaning in their lives (personal and career). Most importantly, we are realizing that we can change the course of our life through our thoughts and attitudes. Trying to be the best you can possibly be speaks highly of your intentions. Intentions are great, but they don't get you there. The psychological foundation of coaching provides coaches with insights into how the mind works and provides them with different strategies to effect lasting changes that will help us fulfill our goals.

Why Nurses Need Coaches

Nurses need coaches for their own personal and professional benefit, as well as to help support their patient care. When a nurse is coached, a light bulb comes on. I know it does for me, whenever I have a coach. When I tell people I have a coach, they look at me in total confusion. They say, "You have a coach?" I have to confirm over and over again that, "Yes, I have a coach!" When people see you from an outside perspective and observe how together you look, they assume that you were probably born into this world perfect and may not realize the work that you have done to achieve your current state. Coaches do not come "ready made." Life, experience, and training make up the coach. It's like the thin runner you see jogging down the street. You might think he or she doesn't need to run, because he or she is so thin. On the other hand, the running could be the very secret to his fit appearance. Coaching is the same way. I often acknowledge that I have the answers within me, but sometimes those answers are hard to access without the help of others. I am accountable to my coach, which is exactly what I need to help maintain that discipline for success.

A coach is also like a hall monitor, in a sense. Coaches ask provocative questions that make you think about your actions and how they relate to what you want in your life. Do you need to do that? Do you need to do this? How does this fit into your current priorities? They aren't glorified busybodies—they are people who are skilled to motivate us and help us reach for goals outside of ourselves. If every nurse had the opportunity to be coached and receive this type of inspiration, the retention and satisfaction of nurses would increase. I can almost guarantee it!

In relation to patients, nurses often feel a great deal of pressure to get patients to do things that realistically they are not able to do. With coaching, you can set your patients up for success by encouraging them to take on one little challenge at a time. The coaching approach is a lot different from psychotherapy and other counseling modalities in which you might give people steps and processes to solve the problems in their lives. Coaching is different because it allows the individual to take charge of his own life, devise his own action plans, and be accountable for his success. Nurses can sometimes take on more responsibility than necessary. The failure of the patient is seen as the failure of the nurse, even when that may be far from the truth. However, by using a coaching model and teaching patients how to take small steps toward change, nurses will probably see a higher success rate. Nurses should explore the coaching model to create a nursing style that is empowering and less enabling. I am not assuming that all nurses are enabling, but because we are nurturers by nature and there are so many of us who are burnt-out, we have to screen for all the possibilities.

The Roots of Coaching

There are many theories in psychology that have been used to create the framework for the coaching models that exist today. In brief, Sigmund Freud planted the seed for us to look to our unconscious mind for answers. Coaches have taken this concept and helped clients to recognize patterns they might not be aware of because they are embedded in the unconscious mind. Bringing these patterns to light helps us progress and move forward. Many clients who seek coaching for spiritual growth and/or to identify their calling in life are approaching (or have passed) middle age. "Carl Jung is probably best known for his theories of ages and stages of life, noting that midlife and beyond (after age 40) most humans begin to search for spiritual meaning, and heed callings for some shift in discovering and then living their life purpose" (Williams, 2008).
"My Personal Story"

A few years ago, if you had mentioned to me that you were working with a life coach, I would have chuckled at you and assumed you had nothing better to do with your money. My kids would call me a "hater." (For those of you who don't have teenagers and aren't accustomed to modern slang, a hater can be defined as a person who resents someone else for doing what he can't, having what he doesn't have, or being what he is not.) I just couldn't justify spending money to have someone to tell me things I should know myself, paying someone to hold my hand because I'm scared to do something new, or having a coach just because it's the trendy thing to do. I was very skeptical because of the large amounts of money that some coaches charge for their services. If people are willing to pay that much, I thought, they deserve what they get. For someone who totally believes in coaching now, I was very critical of the new industry on the horizon.

About 2 years ago, I was sitting at a stoplight twiddling my thumbs. I was en route to my next hospice patient's home. I had made about 9 or 10 visits that day and had begun the process of gathering myself together so that I could be present for the family I was about to visit. I was physically and mentally exhausted. I felt like I couldn't get enough self-care, because it seemed like all my patients were making their transitions at about the same time. I was attending the deaths of several of my patients each week, with little time to grieve, breathe, or nurture myself properly. A little voice inside me helped me make a choice to transition with my patients. Once my last patient transitioned,

I would make a transition myself. I don't believe in coincidences, but my last three patients died during the week I took my certification examination. We all would transition together.

I graduated with a master's degree as a family nurse practitioner in 2004. I had actually completed all my master's coursework about 3 years before that. I would attribute fear and burnout as two significant factors that hindered me from graduating in 2001. My initial research project did not pan out, and I would need to start again. The research project was all that I was lacking to fulfill the requirements for my Master's degree. Sadly enough, I didn't have the motivation to do it. Research, at that time, was something I liked the least and wanted to understand the least. I was intimidated by it and wanted to avoid it at all costs. Of course, I created excuses and then life happened. There seemed to be more reasons to be content where I was and not move forward with my initial plans to become a nurse practitioner. My children needed me, I was burned-out on school and work, and I chose to keep my current job to maintain some stability in my life. I eventually found the motivation to finish my research. When a letter came in the mail that advised me to finish my project or lose all my master's credits, I felt a swift kick in my backside. My graduate advisor, Susan Kasal-Chrisman, rallied and encouraged me off my couch of contentment and worked with me to complete my project. Dr. Judy Beyers, a professor from another university, unknowingly became a powerful coach for me during this time and supported me through the completion of my project. I crossed the scary bridge and that was good enough for me. I had no intentions of taking boards or practicing as a nurse practitioner. Somehow, I had begun to think it was not my path. I was mainly happy that I was able to overcome my fears and achieve closure for finishing something I had started.

The years just flew past. Three years later, I am sitting at a stoplight thinking that I should be doing something different, but hadn't a clue what I could do. My inner voice gently whispered, "FNP." The lightbulb came on. That's it! I would work to find a job as a family nurse practitioner. Then the usual fears set in, because I had been out of school for such a long time. I need to study for boards! I need to pass boards! I had been out of school for 6 years! Panic! Panic! Panic!

Around the time of my transition, I was exploring coaching to enhance my nursing practice. I wanted to combine my master's degree and holistic coaching skills to help improve health care in the community. That's when Linda Bark came into my life. I was seeking ways to become a better coach for my patients, and Linda pointed me inward to a process. She reminded me that I had my own goals to achieve and I, too, was at the dawn of a new horizon. I knew my patients would appreciate the idea that I would be following my path. Before I knew it, I had mapped the preparation plan for my certification exam. I was taken through a series of exercises that allowed me to experience every detail from studying to receiving the final, passing results. It was amazing, because I had no fear. I had so much confidence when I walked in to take the test, the years out of school didn't faze me. I saw my success in the end, and that was the energy I dwelled on. Linda had me visualize the word "pass." She and the coaching group supported me on my "pass" journey. As happy endings go, when the testing machine shut off, the congratulatory message appeared. I couldn't get to my computer fast enough to let Linda know that I had PASSED!

I always believed that coaching is perfect for healthcare settings, because as nurses, we coach our patients all the time. I honor the influence nurses have by serving as resources, guides, and cheerleaders for our patients. Tapping into the coaching aspect for myself was an awakening. I needed to explore coaching fully, before I could formulate an honest opinion about the process. My skepticism was only a minor setback. I was like the little guy in Dr. Seuss's classic book *Green Eggs and Ham*. Sam-I-Am was the little voice inside me urging me to keep an open heart and explore. So I'll have coaching in a box. And I'll have coaching with a fox.

And I'll have coaching in a house. And I'll have coaching with a mouse. And I'll have coaching here and there. Say! I'll have coaching ANYWHERE!

HOLISTIC LIFE COACHING

Holistic life coaching is a means of supporting individuals in fulfilling their specific goals or desires by examining all aspects of their lives and achieving harmony with those aspects. The ultimate reward is the fulfillment, joy, satisfaction, harmony, and the confidence to create and manifest. Holistic life coaching isn't intended to constantly push you to get, get, get, and get more. Holistic life coaching encourages self-awareness so that you have the ability to see the true quality of what you truly want. You can have the desire to be a pink ninja, but a coaching session can help you realize that you only wanted to be a pink ninja because you were being pressured to want that. With that realization, you can make other choices and get on with your "real" life.

The Concept of Coaching

In the coaching process, you have an individual who assumes the role of a facilitator or guide and is skilled in helping to bring out qualities that are hidden deep within you. When you have the desire to accomplish a goal—start a business, learn to dance, improve your singing, exercise, or shed a few pounds—there is a coach out there ready to help you. The coach does not necessarily have to be an expert at what you want to accomplish; however, many people will coach within their area of expertise. The coach's role is not to be a psychotherapist and provide answers for you to solve your problems. The coach's role is to serve as a facilitator and escort you through you own independent journey to accomplish what you desire. I coach in the area of holistic wellness because my background is holistic health and wellness. Some people may coach a person in rose planting, and have never planted a rose before in their life. The beauty of coaching is that you can access resources for your client when necessary.

Coaching can be conducted with individuals or with groups. Group coaching is a useful approach because people can join together and interact with one another in many ways. People within the group can share and serve as resources themselves, because they all represent different walks of life. The individual approach is good too, because you get one-on-one experience with the coach. Both ways serve a purpose.

More and more healthcare professionals are exploring coaching to enhance their practices. As with everything we have discussed in this book, what we share with others is so much more effective when we experience it for ourselves. Holistic coaching is just one aspect of coaching. There is truly a coach for everything. Given the current concerns about the nursing shortage, and nursing surveys that reveal decreased job satisfaction, the support of a coach might prove very helpful. Coaching could be the answer for improving staff retention, resolving conflicts, and increasing job satisfaction.

Reasons to Use a Coach

- Organization
- Self-care
- Establish balance between work and life
- Increase personal productivity
- Teach or improve leadership skills
- Career planning
- Retirement
- Improve and teach communication skills
- Nutritional management
- Weight loss
- Conflict resolution or management
- Management skills and competencies
- Marketing skills
- Health and wellness

Coaching for Self-Care

Nurses can receive benefits from holistic coaching that can help them find direction in their careers or life goals. Coaching can also help nurses incorporate self-care into their personal lives on a daily basis.

Benefits of Coaching for Self-Care

- Self-awareness
- Goal fulfillment
- Empowerment
- Confidence
- Self-improvement
- Career advancement
- Health and wellness
- Abundance
- Peace and harmony

Self-Care Exercise

You can hire a coach anytime you want, but if you aren't truly ready for change, anything you do will probably be a waste of time. Before my experiences with Rebecca and Linda, I had a very brief coaching encounter. I met a wonderful coach who had a great deal to offer me, but I was consumed in a relationship that was emotionally draining and I was working very hard at my job. I was so busy that I did all my homework minutes before our sessions. Eventually, we lost contact with one another and life consumed me. As a matter of fact, so much was going on in my life at that time, I almost forgot that I had even worked with a coach at all. Deep down inside, I know the experience wasn't wasted, but it gave me a greater appreciation for the stages my clients may be in, and how I can support them in those stages. I couldn't appreciate the gift my coach had to offer me at that time.

In my training with Linda Bark, founder of the AsOne Coaching Institute, I was first introduced to the six stages of transition, or change, as described by Dr. James O. Prochaska. The first stage is precontemplation. This stage is when others see the change you need to make, but you are unaware or unwilling to begin the process. Let's determine right now whether you are ready to work with a coach. This brings us to the second stage, which is contemplation. A questionnaire is provided below that can help you determine whether you are ready for an experience with coaching. Don't feel bad if you aren't ready to move forward—this isn't a ploy to make you feel guilty or ashamed. If you do feel like you are ready, you are in the contemplation stage. This stage is described as knowing that you want to make a change, but not knowing how to make it happen. You can move toward readiness by surrounding yourself with supportive and like-minded people who are doing what you desire, or keeping the images of what you desire near your heart. Place pictures around your house so that you don't forget what you want to be when you grow up! This sends a message to your brain that it should be there. There is a catch, however: the universe may take you on a different course. Try not to be so attached to what you are trying to accomplish that you can't recognize that it isn't right for you at this time, if ever. Cinderella's stepsisters did their best to wear her glass slipper, but they couldn't make it fit. I'm not calling you a stepsister (or brother)—I'm just keeping you aware that there is a slipper out there that is your perfect size.

Are You Ready for a Coach?

The following are a list of questions to determine if you are ready for coaching. You must read first each question, then assign each question a ranking from 1 to 10. Write the ranking next to the question. There is a number line to refer to below that will help you to rank each question. For example, I am ready to explore and fulfill my purpose in life. I chose 6 from the number line below. 6 is located under the category of Agree somewhat. This means you are in the middle of being ready to explore and fulfill your purpose in life. Continue answering each question and assigning a ranking number to each. You will be able to determine how much weight each question carries, by the numbers you choose for each question. Tally up the numbers when you have answered all the questions, and determine if you are ready for coaching.

- I am ready to explore and fulfill my purpose in life.
- I am ready to experience harmony in my life.
- I am ready to be accountable to myself.
- I am ready to experience fun, joy, and self-love.
- I am ready to find and live my life's purpose.
- I am ready to relinquish negative self-talk and self-limiting thoughts.
- I am ready to embrace change.
- I am ready to receive abundance and prosperity.
- I am ready for more fun and enjoyment in my life.
- I am ready to explore my interconnectedness with others.

Unnumbered Box 11-1

1	2	3	4	5	6	7	8	9	10
Don't agree			- Agree somewhat -					Totally agree	

<30: This is not the right time for you to try coaching. Determine what is really important to you and meditate on it. Explore your thoughts and remind yourself that you deserve every good thing that comes to you. Be honest with yourself and listen to the inner voice within you.

31–60: The way is open for you to explore coaching for change. The key to your success will be the commitment you make to yourself to take action for what you desire to accomplish and follow through. It would be helpful for you to image what you want to take place and give your energy to that on a daily basis, as you work with your coach.

>60: You have been giving your goal your attention and are ready to begin the work it takes to create it. Meditate and make that call to the coach who feels right to you.

Self-Care Exercise—20 Questions

Let's play 20 questions. If you have ever experienced coaching before, you might have felt that the coach got a tad bit personal. An important part of coaching is asking the client questions to shift his consciousness and bring out what is really inside. You will constantly be asked questions that allow you to explore your intentions, your potential, and your fears. It seems as if coaches often are able to connect with their clients intuitively and push the right buttons, spark the right thought process, and get the creative juices flowing just by asking questions. In this exercise, your job is to answer the question with the first answer that comes to your mind. These answers will no doubt come from a deeper part of your consciousness. When you have completed the questions, give yourself a little break. Come back to the questions every evening for a week, and reread the answers that you have written. See if they hold new meaning for you when you read them. Jot down each new meaning every day in your journal and meditate on them.

20 Questions

1. What does life have in store for you?
2. What do you have in store for your life?
3. What keeps you from being a priority?
4. How do you feel about destiny?
5. How do you feel about fate?
6. Are you in charge of ____?
7. What do you want to know?
8. How did you do it?
9. What is your yearning?
10. What is your passion?
11. What is your urgency in the matter of _____?
12. How many times do you have to _____?
13. How can self-care keep you alive?
14. What have you created at work?
15. What have you created in your relationships?
16. Why is nursing important to me?

17. What is more important than _____ and why?
18. What do you give your joy to?
19. Where are your thoughts?
20. Why do you want _____?

SELECTING A COACH

When selecting a coach of any type, you should consider four factors. The first factor to consider is the coach's training and qualifications. Ask your potential coach the name of the training program he or she has participated in, and then do some exploring online. Most reputable coach training programs have a Web site with detailed information about their program, a directory of coaches, and contact information. The hours of training required for these programs vary from 40 to 150 hours or more. If your coach has 200+ hours of training, there is a good chance he or she has the skills to help you with your life! Many coaching programs are certified through the International Coaching Federation (ICF). When a coach is certified through this association, he or she has completed a certain number of training hours for each level of expertise. The ICF has been around since the late 1990s and sets the standards for coaches professionally and ethically, to ensure that clients receive quality coaching and coaches receive quality training. The ICF also provides a list of coaching programs with which it is affiliated on its Web site.

The second factor is experience. If you choose a coach, make sure his or her background and experience can facilitate your personal growth and progress. Experience is relevant in coaching; however, a coach doesn't have to actually work in your field of expertise to help you. In the Circle of Life process, the coach is instrumental in directing you to the resources you need and relying on the group for support. In other coaching settings, you might be coached by someone who has had experience with what you are currently doing. For example, I coach nurses in the art of self-care because I have firsthand experience with the issues nurses face in the work-force. I can help them deal with these issues and support them appropriately.

The third factor is the degree of professionalism the coach displays in each interaction. What kind of vibe do you get when you talk or connect? If you are waiting for your coach to call at a certain time and he is always late, you might consider coaching him! Does your coach have a business card or did he have to write his number on a piece of paper for you? Does your potential coach have a Web site that you can refer to for information? Does your coach seem frazzled every time you connect? Does your coach badmouth other coaches or coaching models you are considering exploring on your journey? A professional coach will lay things on the line for you in specific terms because she knows that your future is important to you, and so is your time.

The fourth factor to consider is the coach's references. It is always good to have a list of people you can contact and ask about what kind of experience they had with a particular coach. Now, if every reference you call has the coach's last name, there is a good chance he is paying family members to be a reference for him. Don't be afraid to ask for references, because employers do it all the time. You are a consumer and are hiring the coach to provide a service.

Location

As mentioned above, coaching sessions can be conducted individually or in a group setting. Individual coaching sessions can be held in an office, library, coffee shop, or even over the telephone in the comfort of your own home. Because of time zone differences, I have conducted some of my greatest coaching sessions in my pajamas. The possible meeting places are endless and can be anywhere you and your coach decide to meet.

Session Length and Fees

Many coaches will let you have the first session free, as a complimentary introduction to what they can offer you. The prices vary for each coach. The fees are based on the coach's experience and media visibility (a coach who has been on the Oprah Winfrey show will charge more) and the cost of living in your particular area. If the coach you want to work with is a published author, is very visible in the media, and/or has a radio talk show or podcast, you can bet that her fees will reflect that. Some coaches work on a sliding scale to meet the needs of clients who otherwise might not be able to afford coaching. Some coaches will charge for a certain number of sessions as a block, payable in full up front, or they may require you to pay for each session is before it begins. However, most coaches will charge by the month. Prices can range from an average of $75 per coaching session to $350+ per hour or per group of sessions.

Coaching sessions can range from 30 to 90 minutes, depending on the needs of the client. Some coaches offer 15-minute coaching quickies or tune-ups (spot coaching), with enough advance notice (this may or not be included in the coaching fee). Sometimes you can correspond by e-mail or fax, which may or may not be a part of the coaching agreement.

Coaching Contract

Once the coach has made it clear to you what she is able to offer, the next step is to agree upon a contract. Once a verbal agreement has been made to proceed with the coaching, a contract is signed that outlines the expectations of both the client and the coach. They begin the work together, mutually respecting one another and committing to work together in partnership. Both the client and the coach should be very clear about what they expect from each other. Linda

Bark (2009) has suggested some key skills that can help clients benefit from the coaching relationship and achieve their goals. By using these skills, you can be clear about the change you desire and create a plan to arrive at your goal by taking small and steady steps. Before beginning the coaching sessions, the coach should discuss these skills with the client.

- First and foremost, be ready to make a change.
- Be able to cocreate a meaningful partnership with your coach.
- Be able to observe your own behavior.
- Be willing to explore new territory and look at a variety of options.
- Be interested in celebrating your successes.

Other points that should be covered in the contract are timeliness, mutual respect, and payment agreements. The coach and client should also agree on the number of sessions to be conducted and arrange them per month or quarter, or according to project completion. Once the contract is settled, you can move on to the actual coaching.

What a Coaching Session Is Like

A coaching session can be conducted in person and/or over the phone. I find both ways effective. Phone sessions can be beneficial because you can relax in your pajamas if your coach is in a different time zone. However, some people need a face-to-face interaction. This is an important thing to consider when selecting a coach. I have experienced and practiced two different coaching models. I will describe what a typical session in each of these models is like.

Circle of Life Coaching Model

In the Circle of Life coaching model, created by Rebecca McLean and Robert Jahnke, the coach begins by explaining the Circle of Life process. The wonderful thing about the Circle of Life process is that self-care is at the core of the process. There are six phases to explore in this coaching process:

1. Assessing your life—Where do you want to go?
   The coach will help you to look at 12 categories of your life and determine which category you are least satisfied with, so that you can move toward change.

   The 12 categories are:
   1. Life purpose
   2. Self-esteem
   3. Spirituality
   4. Nutrition
   5. Exercise

6. Stress mastery
7. Relationships
8. Finances
9. Work
10. Play
11. Health care
12. Environment

2. Testing your readiness—Are you ready to change?
3. Designing your change—What can I do to make my change happen?
4. Planning your actions—Here are the steps to what I desire to accomplish.
5. Taking action and accessing resources—I am taking action and using different resources to assist me.
6. Reevaluate and revise—I am accountable to my coach and others, and can revise my plan if it doesn't work out like I planned. I can keep doing what I am doing, if it is working to help me achieve my goals.

There are 15 powers of the Circle of Life process that support you in every phase of the process. By understanding each power, you can access the help you need during the coaching process, whenever you need it. The coach will teach you what each of these powers mean and how to use them in your daily life.

1. Self-inquiry and tuning into yourself
2. Acknowledging strengths and weaknesses
3. Readiness for change
4. Group process and testimonial
5. Recognizing challenges
6. Intention and affirmation
7. Setting realistic goals
8. Self-reliance and inner wisdom
9. Targeted action
10. Accountability
11. Expertless system and self-directed
12. Mind/body optimizing practices
13. Acceptance, grace, gratitude, and prayer
14. "Fail safe" system
15. Lifelong learning and continuous improvement

The Circle of Life coach helps you to bring the phases and the power of the Circle of Life together by helping you to identify your strengths, victories, and challenges. There are many different tools you can use to engage your subconscious mind and promote lasting change. Setting your intentions, stating your goals, visualizing your goals achieved, and affirming your goals are just a few things that engage your mind to create the changes you need in your life. The coach helps you create a plan of action for change that is realistic and achievable, not something that is impossible and sets you up for failure and disappointment. The coach also reminds you to keep practicing self-care while trying to achieve your goals, so that you can nurture yourself throughout the process. The coaching process includes a variety of mind/body self-care practices, ranging from tai-chi to breathing exercises that help you develop awareness and conscious relaxation. Once you have learned the process, you can use it to address every issue in your life that you feel you need to change and to achieve your goals (McLean & Jahnke, 2007).

The AsOne Coaching Model

Coaching sessions with an AsOne coach will vary greatly, but in a creative and intuitive way. I have never experienced a coaching process that connects with the individual as intimately as this one does. First, you begin every session with a connection or grounding. I often find myself taking a deep breath whether I am coaching a client or being coached. Linda Bark will ask her clients to give what she calls an "internal weather report," in which they describe how they are feeling in weather terms. Being able to visualize my feelings in this way helps put me in an expansive frame of mind. It puts me in a creative mood, so that I can come up with creative solutions to my challenges. For example, today as I'm writing, I'm feeling "breezy and light."

Coaches use a variety of tools to reach each person's mental processes, because every individual is unique and has different needs. Each coach is trained to use these tools effectively and intuitively, as opposed to trying to fit individuals into a certain way of coaching. Once the coach establishes your nature, he or she can use the tools that will be effective for you.

The AsOne coaching model uses four categories of tools to help create a variety of experiences in each coaching session: Magical, Archaic, Mental, and Mythical. Before the coach chooses which tool to use with you, he or she will ask what if you are interested in trying something new. For example, when I was preparing for my boards, Linda chose to use a Mental tool called the 1 to 10 scale. She asked me if I was interested in standing on a line that ranged from 1 to 10. Standing on number 1 meant that I was not ready to take my boards and standing on 10 meant that I could see myself taking my boards and passing. When I stood on that imaginary line, it was about 1 week before I had to take my exam, and I was at about a 6. I was afraid of failing the exam, because the odds were against me. I had been out of school for so long; I had to bring myself up to speed for the 5 years I hadn't practiced. She asked me if I wanted to try the next number, and I advanced up the line. Then I assessed how that felt and what I could see myself doing to bring me to that point. When I reached the number 7, I was practicing more questions so that I could have the confidence I needed to pass my exam. She gave me the option to advance again, and I went for it. By the time I reached the number 10, my mind had shifted and I was able to see myself passing. Somewhere between 6 and 10, I had decided that I had learned all this stuff before and the most important thing to do now was to denounce fear and make room for the knowledge to flow. I remember that experience like it was yesterday!

Linda also engaged me in some supportive rituals, in the magical category. I plastered the word PASS all over my house, on my computer screensaver, on my cell phone, in my car, and everywhere my brain had an opportunity to be reminded that I was going to pass the exam. Putting PASS on my computer made me have stronger visualizations of passing the computerized test, because I would see PASS on that screen when I was finished. When I did complete my boards, though, I didn't see PASS. I saw a big, fat "Congratulations!" It was so enriching to me to know that I created this experience with my coaching tools. Who knows what the outcome might have been had I not been given these tools to help me visualize success.

During the writing of this book, I had the privilege of having a coaching session with a coaching partner named Fall. She and I have an agreement to coach each other through our coaching practicum over the next few months. I discovered that being new to writing a book made me feel a little insecure and fearful of the unknown. I love holistic nursing and being able to share my knowledge with others, but writing a book is new experience that takes me back to infancy. (And infancy is not always a comfortable stage for us "know-it-all Aquarians!") In our coaching session, Fall used a tool that I had not experienced before. This tool, called dialogue, is from the mythical category and is used when a client is in need of more awareness. For example, Fall asked what I was feeling. I thought I was feeling fear at the time of our session. Fall asked if I could step aside and let fear speak. It seemed silly at the time, but once the voice of fear began to explain its version of the situation to Fall, we learned that insecurity was the emotion that was playing a bigger part in my discomfort. By Fall allowing me to speak from different perspectives within me, I could articulate my feelings out loud and hear what was really going on with these parts of myself. There is something amazing about revealing things deep inside you. Once they come up, you can understand, acknowledge, and move forward. Fall used this dialogue tool so that I could connect with the parts of me that were insecure and fearful, and let my true reality surface. It worked! I was able to identify parts of myself that weren't useful and release them.

All coaching models involve identification of a challenge or change, assessment of readiness, and action plans. I am intrigued by how people can shift their minds to create the expansion they need for change. We can do many amazing things when our adrenaline is rushing, such as lifting a car off a person or rescuing an animal from oncoming traffic. We do what we have to do because the moment calls for it, and we don't have time to argue with our own "I can't" or "I shouldn't" thoughts. To be able to tap into our hidden potential and achieve something without being forced to by a crisis is an amazing thing. There are many ways to get there, and they can be as simple as purchasing a planner or reading Angel Cards. We just have to be open to the "how" and the "there."

BECOMING A COACH

The best place to find a coach is the same place you would find a coaching program. The ICF has a number of resources for both coaches and clients seeking a coach. You can explore its Web site and learn about the requirements and standards of coaching, and the variety of coaching programs out there to suit your needs. You can also learn about the different levels of credentials coaches can achieve.

There are many good coaching programs out there. I mentioned the Circle of Life and AsOne Coaching Institute above, not to promote one coaching program over all the others, but because I've had personal (and amazing) experiences with them. You will do an injustice to yourself if you invest money in a program you haven't researched, thinking you can simply take someone's word about it. Coaching programs are not "one size fits all." I am a hospice nurse by profession, and the thought of being a grief coach was appealing to me. But I found myself migrating to something else. See how that works for you. In the famous words of Smokey Robinson and the Miracles, "My momma told me, you better shop around!"

REFERENCES

Bark, L. (2008). *AsOne coaching manual*. Alameda, CA: AsOne Coaching Institute.

Bark, L. (2009). *Wholist coaching: A new way of coaching...a new level of success and fulfillment*. Alameda, CA: Not yet published.

McLean, R., & Jahnke, R. (2007). *The Circle of Life participant guide book. The Circle of Life: A personal health action, self-empowerment system*. Santa Barbara, CA: Health Action.

Williams, P. (2008). Coaching evolution: From psychological theory to applied behavorial change. *Psychology Alliance*, 19–22.

SUGGESTED READING LIST

Stoltzfus, T. (2006). Finding the right coach for you. *Coach, 22*, 1–2.

Williams, P. (2004). Coaching evolution and revolution: The history, development, and distinctions that will define coaching as the most organizational development of the future. *Absolute Advantage*, 7–9.

Williams, P. (2006). The evolving profession of life coaching. *Personal Fitness Professional Magazine*, 1–3.

Williams, P. (2007). Coaching from the inside-out. *Psychology Alliance, 5*(2), 41–42.

Williams, P. (2009). The theoretical foundations of coaching. *Choice, 4*(2), 49–50.

CHAPTER 12

Four Spiritual Practices for Self-Care

RACHEL Y. HILL

"Prayer is exhaling the spirit of man and inhaling the spirit of God."
—EDWIN KEITH

INTRODUCTION TO FOUR SPIRITUAL PRACTICES FOR SELF-CARE

A book on self-care would not be complete without discussing ways to incorporate spirituality into this process. We can meet our physical needs by resting, exercising, practicing good nutrition, and getting a massage every month. We can meet our mental needs by keeping a journal, taking classes for growth, and reading books. But we must also give attention to the spiritual being that exists within all of us. All of these aspects of ourselves must be maintained in balanced proportions for us to achieve the harmony we desire. It is very easy to neglect the spiritual being, because it doesn't cough, bleed, or break out in a visible rash requiring immediate medical attention. However, failing to recognize the signs of spiritual needs can prove to be very devastating in the long run. Nurses are at risk of experiencing spiritual distress in many healthcare settings. Settings where traumas are witnessed repeatedly, hospice settings where patients are cared for during their transition, neonatal units where infants struggle for their lives, and mental health units where mental disease has overcome the realities of men and women can be the breeding grounds that create a spiritual drain on the nurses who are providing care. Once that nurse finds he or she is unable to answer a patient's question, meet a patient's needs, or provide hope to a family member, he or she begins to look inward for answers. There is a possibility that no answers will be found, because there is no substance left to draw from. If she is not in a position of self-awareness, her answers may come from a place of dismay and disillusionment.

There are four powerful tools that support our spiritual existence as human beings: prayer, meditation, affirmation, and gratitude. These spiritual tools can help us connect to our Creator, our inner selves, and the dreams and desires we wish to accomplish here on Earth. The beauty of these spiritual tools is that each one can be practiced outside of any religious affiliation or in conjunction with any religious practice. These spiritual practices have been used for hundreds, if not thousands, of years, and each one has its own particular lineage. Many people believe that we are spirit first; therefore, when we are able to connect with our own souls and the souls of others, we experience a natural state of interconnectedness and being.

PRAYER

Not everyone is comfortable sharing his or her spiritual practices with others, and that is okay. The first time a patient asked me to pray with her, I hesitated and asked, "Really? You really are wanting me to pray to God with you?" She looked confused, but I adjusted quickly because I knew she was depending on me. We held each other's hand and began to pray.

Common Terms Related to Prayer

Conversational prayer – Communication with a higher power, in a form that has no structure and covers an array of topics from forgiveness to gratitude.

Intercessory prayer – Communication with a higher power to ask for help or support for someone else.

Meditative prayer – Communion with a higher power in a quiet way, reflecting sensitivity to the presence of that higher power.

Petitional prayer – Communion with a higher power in relation to a need or concern for spiritual or material help or guidance.

Ritual prayer – Communion with a higher power in a form that is memorized and recited by individuals or groups.

Prayer – Individual or group communion with a higher power.

Prayer is what I know as talking to God. Does prayer work or not? Researchers are finding more information every day about the impact of prayer in the healthcare setting. Prayer before surgery, distance prayer for others, healthcare professionals praying before they carry out procedures or begin their day in the clinic are just a few examples I have personally experienced. I have often wondered how prayer works. I believe in a higher power, and I also believe in the Universal Law of Attraction. I have observed that when we place our attention on something for a certain length of time, coupled with a strong faith, we can shift our reality to accommodate our needs and desires. Our higher guidance, angels, and conscious and subconscious minds all get involved to shift our reality and make things so. This chapter isn't about teaching you to pray. Prayer is very personal for each individual, and my way may not work for you (and vice versa). This chapter is meant to serve as a friendly reminder that you have this resource available to you wherever you go and whenever you need it.

Prayer is a common practice for many religions all over the world. Christianity, Judaism, Islam, Buddhism, Sikhism, and Hinduism all use prayer as a spiritual modality (Farah & McColl, 2008). Prayer is a spiritual practice that connects us to our Creator or higher guidance. Not every nurse has a belief in a higher power. Not every nurse is affiliated with a particular religion in conjunction with his or her spiritual practices. However, prayer is a resource that is used by many people. According to Farah and McColl (2008), there are four types of prayers that are most commonly used by Americans: conversational prayer, meditative prayer, petitional prayer, and ritual prayer. The majority of Americans offer conversational prayers, or prayers that have no structure and are a direct communication with God. In this type of prayer, we thank God for blessings, talk to God in our own words, ask God for forgiveness, and seeking guidance for making decisions. The second most common type of prayer among Americans is meditative prayer, which involves sitting quietly and focusing on the presence of God, worshipping and adoring God, and listening to God. Third is petitional prayer, which is used to ask for help in times of need. Last in this group are ritual prayers, which involve the memorization of prayers or passages from books.

My Personal Experience with Prayer

I have done my share of praying during my lifetime. With my grandfather being the pastor of a church, there was always a weekly prayer service I had to attend. In these services, people would kneel at the altar or in their pews. I could hear many of the members praying outwardly, asking God for things, praying for other people, or even thanking him for the things they had been blessed with. Being a little girl, I found myself in a deep observation and confusion when I would hear adults praying these long prayers about God, any, and everything. I had no clue how I was supposed to pray to get through to God. I would often wonder if I needed to use big words, if I needed to ask for certain things in a special order, or what happens if I ask for too much? The process of prayer seemed more complicated than what I could comprehend. I figured it would make sense to me when I became an adult. However, it happened much sooner for me than I thought it would. Aside from praying for an Easy-Bake Oven, saying my prayers at night, and blessing my food, I never had a reason to pray as a child. Life was carefree for me and I was oblivious to the cares of the world. One day my cousin Vaughn suddenly developed Guillain-Barré syndrome. He was 9 years old and completely lost the use of his legs. The entire community and members of neighboring churches began to pray every day and night for his recovery. I was worried, but I organized my prayer so that I could reach God too.

I was about 10 and suddenly very much aware of my mortality, knowing that my cousin could die from this illness.

Within days after Vaughn became ill, his 6-year-old brother, Chris, also grew very ill, but he did not seem to have the same symptoms. The church members joined in prayer for him, hoping that the doctors would find out what was wrong and that the parents would stay strong in faith. Chris was having abdominal pain, which eventually was diagnosed as a ruptured appendix. This caught my attention. I could see the stress on my aunt and uncle's faces; they knew their two sons were facing death, and there was nothing they could do but wait. It was during this period that I found a purpose for praying, and I prayed for them every minute. I held to my deep belief that things would be all right. Chris had emergency surgery, and the surgeon was tremendously puzzled by what he found. The doctor told my aunt that when they opened my cousin's abdomen, the pockets of poison in his body had walled themselves off in sacs and were completely contained.

The two brothers were able to leave the hospital together. They were able to attend a church service together. The congregation had been praying for them for so long; the boys wanted to take the opportunity to say hello to the church members and thank them for their prayers and support. My cousin Vaughn asked the church to keep praying for him so that he could walk again. Guess what? The church members decided to pray for him right then and there, again. He took the first four steps immediately after they prayed, in front of the congregation. From that day on, Vaughn's health improved and he went on to participate in many basketball championships, received many sports scholarships, and won many track and field awards. Both brothers are miracles and a true reflection of what prayer can do.

In the course of nursing and practicing self-care, we don't always remember to pray when we need it. Sometimes we find it very difficult to pray for ourselves because it seems irrelevant to our existence. We may think, "What good will prayer really do? Things are too far gone for prayer to help now." But if a patient needs prayer, I know that I am now willing to pray for him or her instantly and on demand, and feel comfortable doing so. When I am having a problem, sometimes prayer can be a delayed reaction. I catch myself and think, "I need to pray about this one!" I tend to pray in the morning before I start work, so that I can channel my energy toward being open to the many possibilities for growth and for handling any challenge with grace and ease. I pray when there are conflicts in the workplace among coworkers, patients, family, and friends. I will pray a petitional prayer, because I desire a specific outcome to be met. I want the relationship to be restored to balance, so that the work environment can remain healthy and balanced. If it doesn't seem like it is working, I go into my freestyle mode, which is the conversational format mentioned earlier. I am seeking guidance because I don't have a clue about what is going on in the current situation and what

I should do. I ask for help from the universe so that I can plant the seed in my mind that I am loved, supported, and capable of great things.

What Are the Benefits of Prayer?

Prayer can provide an overall improved sense of well-being. People who pray tend to have faith. Faith is a part of positive thinking and expecting that the best situation will present itself. Prayer has a calming effect, because we release what we accept we can't accomplish on our own. We turn it over to a higher power than ourselves. I was talking to a coworker who had been trying to have a baby for quite some time. She and her husband had tried for 7 or 8 years, to the point of frustration. She said that they had decided to let it go; they were fine with the child they had, and took responsibility for their future happiness. She and her husband purchased a new house, she got a new job, and 2 months later, she found out she was pregnant. We laughed because despite all the effort you can put into making something work, sometimes it's better to just step away from the situation. "Let go and let God" is what I always say!

Prayer Exercises for Self-Care

If you haven't prayed in a while, these self-care exercises will get you back into the swing of things. We will start by simply incorporating prayer back into our lifestyle. It doesn't take a great deal of time to do these exercises. We can attach prayers to activities we already do, so it can become a habit or a ritual for us. These self-care exercises will definitely take you back!

Bedtime prayer

Do you remember when you were a little kid and would get on your knees and say your prayers before you went to bed every night? "Now I lay me down to sleep, I pray to the Lord my soul to keep, if I should die before I wake, I pray to the Lord my soul to take. God bless Mommy, God bless Daddy, and God bless Grandma Jo." If you have long since stopped saying your prayers before you go to bed, this is a perfect opportunity for you to begin again. There is something magical about making the last thing you do before you sleep sacred and special. That is what prayers are. They are sacred messages that never die; once they leave our lips, they exist forever. The last thought you have before sleeping will revolve around your connection to your higher power and your connection with yourself and others. If there is a problem or issue you are experiencing, you can sleep on it. Who knows? You may get your answer back in the form of a beautiful dream or wake to find that you have a different mindset about the situation. Nevertheless, your prayer has been put out into the universe and you can begin to draw the support you need to help the situation work out for the highest good.

Grace or blessing your food

Here is another exercise taken from my early childhood that I still manage to do to this day. It is a simple prayer that I say over my food before I eat. You may remember the prayer, "God is good, God is great, let us thank him for our food! Amen." You may also remember those long, elaborate prayers that Uncle Tommy recited before holiday meals, when all you wanted to do was eat, but he wouldn't stop praying! This isn't like that at all. Since you have to eat every day for your nourishment, how about giving a prayer of thanks for your food and blessing it before it enters your body? Sounds simple enough.

Work-shift prayer

Here is an exercise that I just recently took up myself: praying before the work shift begins and praying after it ends. There is something amazing about the harmony this activity has created for me. I'm not saying that every day goes perfectly when I pray. But the workday seems much more tolerable and easier to manage, regardless of what takes place. It is like I have sprinkles of grace all over everything, helping me to get through my day peacefully and efficiently. The prayers I pray at work go from the top to the bottom. I pray for the CEOs and the decisions they make regarding the staff and patient care. I pray for the staff to make the wisest decisions for the patients and themselves. I pray for the CNAs, physical and occupational therapists, and even the janitorial staff. No one gets left out, but I feel like I have a connection with everyone and we are all on this shift for a reason and a purpose. I am open to whatever that lesson may be. Once that shift is over and I am going home, I say my prayers for the day to resolve itself without difficulty. If there is anything that was left undone, I ask for the strength to manage it. I also begin to shift my role to that of mother, sister, friend, neighbor, significant other, etc., and pray that I can enjoy my family fully and leave work at the door.

If you aren't an active prayer, consider incorporating these prayers into your life. Experience how this ritual works for you. How does your workday go when you pray before you begin? How quickly are conflicts resolved at work when you pray about them? How well do you rest at night since you have started praying? How does your food taste, since you now bless it? Write about your observations in your journal. Next, you can begin incorporating more prayer into your life. When a coworker is grumpy or angry, you can choose to pray for him or her instead of engaging in gossip or criticism. When you see an ambulance go by, you can say a prayer for the highest good to be done in the situation for all involved. You can pray for your family when you are unable to be with them because of work. You can pray for your coworkers when you are not on the clock.

MEDITATION

"Meditation is the tongue of the soul and the language of our spirit."
—JEREMY TAYLOR

The most important thing a person can do for himself or herself is to meditate. People have an amazing number of thoughts in their minds every second, and the world we live in reflects the quality of our thoughts. Meditation is the best way to quiet all the chatter we are experiencing and allow us to hear God. I definitely can tell the difference when I am meditating. I can see how I am reflected in everyone I come in contact with. I have learned that there is always a way out of difficult situations. Recently I have found myself in difficult situations that I could have dealt with by being dishonest, but instead I prayed for an honest way to resolve the situation and it appeared. Hallelujah! I feel myself becoming a better parent and being able to learn more, and more quickly, because of my ability to concentrate. I do have times when discipline is an issue, and I pray for the strength to make wise spiritual choices that serve my higher mind, and to have wisdom in my relationships with my children, family, friends, coworkers, and patients.

Meditation is what I know as listening to what God has to say to me. Meditation is another ancient art that goes back as far into history as prayer, affirmation, and the art of gratitude. Put simply, when you meditate, you focus your attention on your breathing rhythm or on an image, word, or sound. The purpose of meditation is to quiet the mind, which can be very active with thoughts and chatter in today's busy society. "Do this now, do this later, be here, be there, answer this call light, change this dressing, call this doctor, and call this pharmacy!" YIKES! It takes some definite awareness to have peace of mind these days. The mental chatter can be so overwhelming that it is a challenge to hear the still voice deep inside that provides us with guidance and direction.

I used to consider myself a "bootleg" meditator, because I didn't know the formal terms for the things I was doing to become still within. I always thought that meditation consisted of sitting on the floor with your legs crossed and your hands in some distorted configuration. I didn't know that when I was performing the 36-breaths exercise in my Jin Shin Jyutsu practice, I was meditating. When I would go out to my car, turn on my music, and focus on the sound of the flute, or when I would walk around the hospital and observe the air on my face, I was in meditation. I used to pick a word that would support me and repeat it over and over and over again, until it seemed like the word and I were dancing together. Little did I know I was experiencing stillness, mindfulness, breathing, mantras, and mudras, all of which are the special ingredients in various forms of meditation. Now that I am more educated on the subject, I still receive the same benefits—I just have descriptions and terms that I can use to make more sense to others than just saying, "I want you to breathe like this and put your hands like that." However, even though I've learned a lot about meditation, and some helpful terms, I will always consider myself a lifelong student.

Common Terms Related to Meditation

Breathing – The act of respiration, taking air into the lungs to supply the body with oxygen, and releasing carbon dioxide to cleanse the body of waste and purify the blood.

Concentrative meditation – Meditating on a focal point, such as a sound or object, or chanting mantras to develop concentration and awareness.

Mantras – Mantras are words of power that have a mental, physical, and spiritual impact and are used as tools for meditation.

Meditation – Meditation is the practice of stilling the mind.

Mindfulness meditation – Mindfulness meditation is meditating by focusing on the breath as a point of concentration.

Mudras – Hand positions of power that have mental, physical, and spiritual impacts on individuals and are used as tools for meditation.

Stillness – A state of quietness that clears the mind of mental chatter, allowing an individual to hear his or her inner guidance.

Types of Meditation

There are two basic types of meditation. The first type of meditation is concentrative meditation. In this form of meditation, we learn to develop the skill of focusing our attention, generally on an object, a sound, a word, or a sacred phrase that has a spiritual purpose (mantra). Through this focused attention, we develop the skill of concentration and self-discipline, which allows us to control our mental chatter and accomplish many amazing things. Candle flames, leaves, and water droplets are examples of points of focus for meditative exercises.

The second form of meditation is called mindfulness meditation, which is the simple act of focusing our attention on our breath. Monitoring the breathing process puts us in tune with our body and sensations related to breathing. As we practice more, we develop a deeper experience of our immediate presence, our surroundings, our emotions, and sounds. Mindfulness meditation is the best medicine for helping us stay in the here and now (the "here and now" being the very breath we are breathing at this moment). The breath comes with the inhalation and fades with the exhalation. Each breath is symbolized as an opportunity to begin anew, which offers a sense of peace for the meditator. The experience also allows us to realize that nothing lasts forever, but there is always a rebirth in some form or another. "Mindfulness meditation is basically a life-affirming process in which individuals are asked to continually return to the physical sensation of breath (life) moving in and out of the body. This process requires individuals to set aside their usual and familiar ways of being in the world" (Ott, 2004).

I used to have a hard time understanding this concept of the "here and now." People were always telling me to "be one with the moment, be one with universe, be one with your emotions, be one, be one, be one." I would say to myself, "Enough already!" I thought they were pompous gurus just giving me one more hoop to jump through before I could reach enlightenment. With a little time and repeated meditation, I calmed down. I realized that the only times I hurt in my life were when I was digging through my past dirty laundry or was overwhelming myself with the possibilities of what had not yet happened. The only place I could actually be safe and secure was where I was. I was missing that totally.

When I was a little girl, I would watch my sister keep a pack of bubble gum forever (or what seemed to me like forever). She worried so much about using it all up and not having any left for later that she couldn't bring herself to actually chew the gum. I, on the other hand, would end up chewing the whole pack in a day, feeling bad about my lack of discipline the whole time because I knew I should try to save some. I don't think either of us were really able to have the fullest experience with our bubble gum because of our extremes. I recognized what "being present" meant for me and what my guru friends were trying to relate to me. When I recognized the truth, the pain left. I read about my experience of clarity when I began to study Buddhism and other religions. I realized that this was not a new revelation by any means, and other people have figured this out. Eckhart Tolle wrote an amazing book called the *Power of Now*. In this book, he talks about presence and living in a meditative way so that we can be fully engaged in our experiences. This is where the real power is in our lives, and meditation can help facilitate this growth.

What Are the Benefits of Meditation?

Nurses can benefit greatly from incorporating meditation into their lifestyles because it can help connect them to their higher wisdom and guidance. "Deepening the awareness of ourselves through practices of meditation can change the way we respond to the world and the way we respond to others—including patients—for the better" (Wright, 2007). We will have good days and bad days at home and at work, but meditation helps us to see those days as neutral. We learn to treat them all the same, because we know they won't last forever. We are not detached from the world or our emotions, but we see our emotions and temporary situations for what they are. We take on a more expansive view of what is occurring in our world. A significant benefit of meditation is deep relaxation, which contributes to stress relief, clarity, insight, increased immune function, and much more. "By directing attention away from worries about the future or preoccupation with the past, meditation reduces stress, a major contributing factor in many health problems" (Anonymous, 2002).

Meditation Exercises for Self-Care

Kundalini Meditation

The following self-care exercises will give you a basis to start your meditative practice.

We discussed Kundalini yoga in a previous chapter. Since meditation is an important component of yoga, we will explore it in more detail now. There are five components to Kundalini yoga meditation, as described by Hari Kaur Khalsa (2006) in *A Woman's Book of Meditation*:

1. Seated meditation posture
2. Breathing pattern
3. Mudras
4. Eye focus
5. Mental focus (a mantra or visualization)

Seated Meditation Posture

Meditation has a profound impact on many systems of the body. Your endocrine system and nervous system are stimulated. Keeping your spine straight allows for a clear flow of energy. You can sit in a chair with your back straight (not touching the chair) in chair pose or lay on your back with your knees supported. Another suggested pose for meditation is the easy pose (Sukhasana), or sitting on the floor with your legs crossed. Figure 12-1 illustrates the easy pose. I like to sit on a sheepskin mat or a blanket or cushion when I meditate, because it insulates me. Meditation can increase your sensitivity to temperature changes. If getting down on the floor is a challenge for you, you can sit in a chair. This seated position is called the Egyptian pose and is illustrated in Figure 12-2. This position requires you to sit on a chair with your back away from the chair back, spine straight, and feet flat on the floor. Your hands rest in your lap, palms facing upward.

Breathing Pattern (Pranayam)

Long, deep yogic breathing (from Kundalini yoga)

Begin each breath through the nose. The nose serves as a filter of the air. It warms the air we breathe in and acts as a natural humidifier. When the air is taken into our body through the nose, it is balanced as it enters. The left

Figure 12-1   Easy pose seated meditation position.

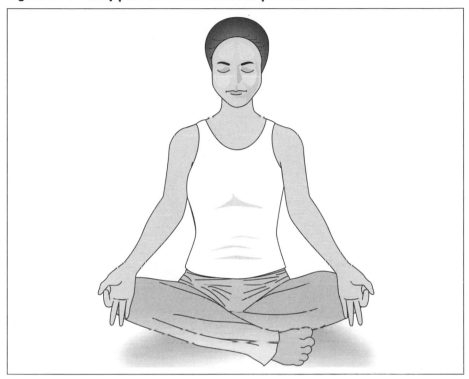

nostril represents our female energy and the right nostril represents our mascu-line energy. This is how the air should always enter our bodies.

Inhale.

Start by pushing the navel point outward and begin filling the lungs with breath from the abdomen upward.

Exhale.

To exhale completely, release as much "leftover" air as possible.

Segmented breathing

This breathing technique can help you manage your moods and is good for bringing refinement to your breathing. Take some long, deep yogic breaths first. You can sit cross-legged on the floor or in a chair with your back straight. As you inhale your first breath, break the breath up in four equal segments. An easy way to break the breath up is to sniff four times, in equal parts. Hold the breath out for a few seconds. Inhale in four equal segments or four equal

Figure 12-2   Egyptian pose chair seated meditation position.

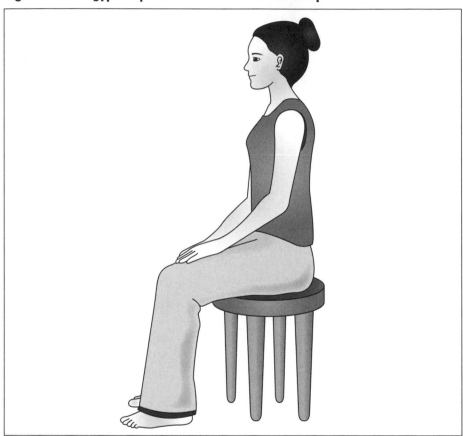

sniffs, and exhale in four equal segments or four equal sniffs. To complete the process, take in four equal segments of breath, and release one long, continuous breath. This type of breathing can increase your clarity and mental concentration, helps to strengthen you, and helps you manage your mental and emotional being.

Mudras

Mudras are special hand and arm postures or holds that achieve a certain purpose. These are also referred to as energetic seals because they circulate energy in the body that helps you achieve a certain level of healing on different levels of your being. Mudras are used for different purposes. They can relax and they can

Figure 12-3   Gyan mudra hand position.

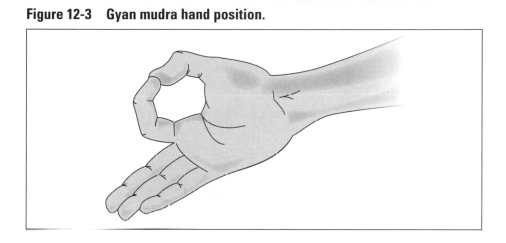

also revitalize. Different meditations use different mudras in conjunction with them. The most common mudra I use is the Gyan Mudra (represents knowledge and expansion), which is illustrated in Figure 12-3.

Gyan Mudra: Place the tip of your thumb together with the tip of your index finger. This stimulates knowledge and ability.

Eye Focus

During meditation, the eyes can be kept focused on certain positions to stimulate and cause different effects to occur. There are five common points of eye focus, as described by Hauri Kaur Khalsa (2006). These positions are the Third Eye point, the Lotus point, the Moon Center, the Crown Chakra point, and the One-Tenth Open point. For our purposes, we will practice two of the five: the Third Eye point (illustrated in Fig. 12-4) and the Crown Chakra point (illustrated in Fig. 12-5).

The Third Eye point or brow point

At the top of your nose, between your eyebrows, is your brow point. Your pituitary gland is also here at this point. To focus on the Third Eye point, you simply bring your attention to it, with your eyes gently raised. The benefits of focusing on this point increased intuition and foresight, and stimulation of the pituitary gland.

The Crown Chakra

When you on the top of your head with your eyes closed, you are focusing on the Crown Chakra point. This position can connect your with your higher

Figure 12-4   Third eye point.

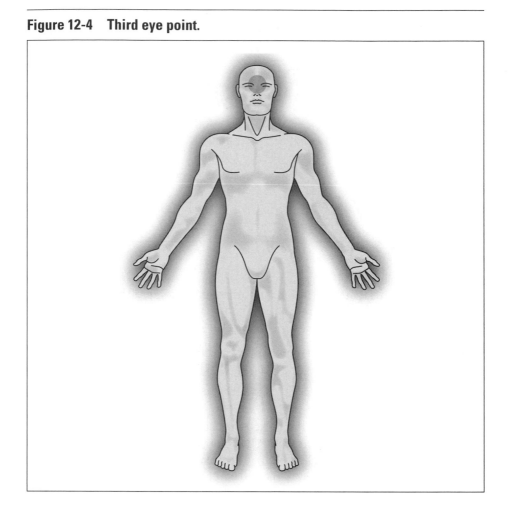

guidance, your Creator, and the universe. This is an expansive point of focus that enables you to become bigger than yourself.

Mantras

When you chant a mantra, you are using sound to impact your conscious mind. This grouping of words or sounds creates a current that can control your mental vibration and provide a purpose or direction for your mind to take. We have discussed the power of words throughout different chapters in this book. Mantras are another example of how words are used to send out a message to the universe in an effort to create the effects of what we desire or meditate on.

Figure 12-5   Crown chakra point.

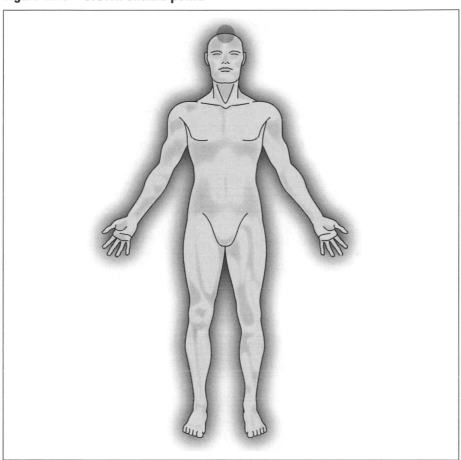

Sat Nam (Bij Mantra)

The Sat Nam is a mantra I have incorporated into my life since I began my yoga training. I always end each yoga class by chanting this mantra. This mantra is similar to Namaste. Many yogic and spiritual practices will place their palms together close to the heart and bow saying "Namaste." This is an acknowledgment of the spirit in each of us. The God in me acknowledges the God in you. The spirit in me acknowledges the spirit in you. Sat Nam is carried out in a similar fashion. It means "The Truth is your identity; God's name is the truth." I answer the telephone this way, say hello and goodbye this way, and end my e-mails this way.

Example of a complete Kundalini yoga meditation

Seven-Wave "Sat Nam Meditation"
Sit in easy pose. Place your palms flat together at the center of your chest, with your thumbs touching the center of the sternum. With your eyes closed, look up slightly, focusing on the brow point or the point between both eyes. Inhale deeply, concentrating on your breath. With the exhale, chant the mantra in the law of seven or the law of the tides. When you perform the Sat Nam meditation in the law of the tides, you are vibrating Sat six times. An example of this is Sa-a-a-a-a-a, with the last sound being tnam. You are simply vibrating "Sat" into six waves or parts, and letting the last sound "Nam" be the seventh wave. On each wave, visualize yourself sending the sound through each of the chakras like a thread. Sat begins at the first chakra at the rectum. As you work your way up through each chakra, pull the sound through the physical area it corresponds to.

First center: the rectum (Sa)

Second center: the sex organs (a)

Third center: the navel point (a)

Fourth center: the heart (a)

Fifth center: the throat (a)

Sixth center: the brow point (a)

Seventh center: the top of the head (tnam)

In this meditation, you activate the energy of the mind that erases and establishes habits. This is good for new yoga students, to open them up to new experiences, continue the exercise for 15 minutes.

Here is the breakdown of the meditation so that you can see how the various components of meditation come together (Fig. 12-6).

1. Seated meditation posture: Easy pose.
2. Breathing pattern: Inhale deeply, concentrating on the breath. With the exhale, chant the mantra in the law of seven or the law of the tides. Vibrate "Sat" in six waves, and let "Nam" be the seventh wave.
3. Mudras: Hands are in prayer pose.
4. Eye focus: Brow point.
5. Mental focus: A mantra or visualization.
   Mantra: Vibrate "Sat" in six waves, and let "Nam" be the seventh wave.
   Visualization: On each wave, thread the sound through the chakras, beginning at the first chakra, which is the rectum. As you work your way up through each chakra, let the sound radiate through the physical area it corresponds to.

Figure 12-6   Seated meditation position.

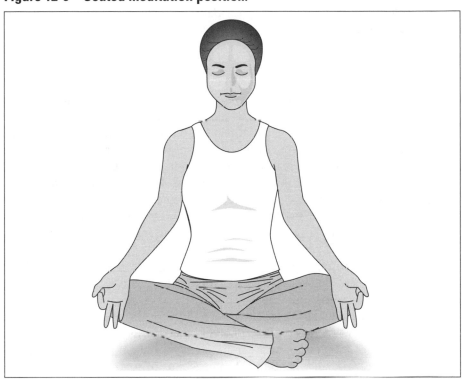

Mindfulness Meditation

Mindfulness meditation is simple. All you need to do is find a comfortable place to sit, where you can be relaxed and your spine can be straight and aligned from the base of your spine to the top of your head. Your feet should be planted flat on the floor with palms resting in your lap, facing upward. You can also sit on the floor in easy pose, with your legs crossed and hands resting in your lap. Keep your eyes gently closed and begin focusing your attention on your breath. Experience each breath as it comes into your nose and out through your nose. Feel the fall and rise of your chest. Feel your belly as it expands and contracts also. Feel reverence for your breath, because it will never return to you again. Feel reverence and gratitude for each breath, because you don't know when it will be your last one. Keep your attention focused on the breath. If your thoughts wander, gently bring yourself back to your breath in a gentle and loving way (Ott, 2004).

AFFIRMATION

"You will be a failure, until you impress the subconscious with the conviction you are a success. This is done by making an affirmation which "clicks."
—FLORENCE SCOVEL SHINN

Affirmations activate our prayers and reinforce the guidance we receive through our meditations. An affirmation is a statement of purpose in which an individual speaks with the intention to manifest that statement into his or her existence. Every word we speak about others and ourselves is put out into the universe, never to be returned to us. Each word we speak is a perfect opportunity for us to manifest our words into reality. Affirmations help us to be conscious of what we speak, because we are speaking with a purpose. Just as we eat a healthy balanced diet to have healthy and strong bodies, we speak positive words to create a strong and healthy life (or reality). If someone gives you a compliment and tells you that your jeans are flattering to you, how do you respond to him or her? Do you say, "With these fat old thighs? Pretty soon I'll have to lie on the bed to get my butt into these things!" or do you say, "Thank you so much! I was thinking the same thing when I looked at myself in the mirror today!"? (Okay, the second statement might be a little extreme, but it is by far a better comment.)

According to the law of attraction, we attract what we give our attention to. Affirmations are a perfect example of the law of attraction in motion. When we ponder, dwell, meditate, even worry, we are giving our attention to some form of thoughts that contain some content that impacts us in some way. The degree of attention you give your thoughts attracts a certain degree of attention from outside sources. Try thinking that you can't wait to go to work to see your patients. This thought can be so strong that when you arrive, your patients will be excited that you are with them for that shift. Your coworkers will be energetic and welcoming to you. You will have created a wonderful workday simply by directing your thoughts.

Now, if you dislike your job, your patients, and the people you work with, we face a bit of a challenge. Affirmations are a wonderful solution to this dilemma. Since your thoughts are probably not focused on what you want to happen, it will be necessary to shift them there. Think about what you want to take place first. Say, "I love my job, my patients, and the people I work with." Affirmations are phrases that we speak based on thoughts we think, and may or may not be true for us at that particular moment. It doesn't matter if the affirmation is not true, for now. You can "fake it till you make it!" What is important is that you are shifting your thoughts from what you don't want to what you do want. This allows the law of attraction to work.

A simple statement can have such a profound impact on your life and your ability to create your reality. Eventually, your conscious mind and your subconscious mind will agree, and you will see the outcome that you desire. As long as your affirmations are based on realistic thoughts and you are completing the actions needed on your part to move the situation forward, you will have the ingredients for success. For example, you can say, "I am the best cardiac nurse in the world!" This is a good affirmation because you have the potential to be the best cardiac nurse in the world. But you cannot say "I am the best cardiac nurse in the world" if you haven't even enrolled in nursing school yet. You have to backtrack and give your brain a picture it can adjust to. Affirm that you will get into nursing school, and then affirm that you will graduate from the program; then you will be much closer to affirming that you are the best nurse in the world. Even if you are already a nurse, the affirmation will not come true for you if you don't read and study about the cardiac cycle, attend classes, pursue continuing education opportunities, and work in a cardiac setting where you can maximize your ability to excel at what you desire. It takes action to bring affirmations to life. Just saying an affirmation is not enough to create change within our lives, our jobs, and our relationships with others. However, it is a start.

How Do Affirmations Work?

Affirmations are phrases of power that help direct our lives. Listen to a person's words and you can get a good picture of where his or her thoughts are. Affirmations are mental and spiritual tools that allow us to take control of a life we may feel we have little control over. It's true that there are things that are beyond our control, but with affirmations we have more of the rope in the game of tug-of-war. We can handle the things we are unable to control much better because we are grounded and have solid footing. We can find the lessons and continue to affirm our truth regardless of what the world says or looks like. It is easy to choose to sit around and say, "Life is hard, work is hard, my patients are crazy, my boss is really crazy, etc." Life plays out exactly as you speak it, in most cases. Negative talk is of no service to you in the long run, especially if you can't learn from your experiences and make your talk affirming and positive. Affirmations are the switch that takes you off of autopilot and allows you to take conscious responsibility for your thoughts, your words, and the eventual actions you will create through your thoughts.

Let's do a little experiment and put our words to the test. Take a deep breath and say, "I am really very tired." Now explore how you feel after saying it. How do you feel? Tired and drained? Next, say aloud to yourself, "I am supercharged and ready for action!" How does that phrase feel to you? Do you feel more energized and less heavy than when you were tired? It is amazing what your words and mind can accomplish together. My son Chandler often gets tired when he has to do the dishes in the evening. He doesn't know how he will muster up the strength to get his chores done. Once I mention going for frozen custard when he gets done, his tune changes and he is moving faster than lightning.

Affirmations are spiritual tools and mental tools all in one. I think they begin as mental seeds that blossom into big bean stalks that reach into the heavens. Once you plant them, they take on a life of their own. Affirmations are mental exercises, at first, because they are spoken consciously and openly. The conscious mind knows what we should be doing and what we should be, but it doesn't always have the motivation or strength to make it happen. Your conscious mind knows that affirmations are beneficial. With affirmation, you are attempting to engage your subconscious mind. The subconscious mind has a desire to give you whatever you want. It just sits back and watches your every conscious move. It watches what you do and say, wondering if you are really serious about what you are saying. After you have established a pattern in which you speak what you desire while you are putting action toward achieving that desire, your subconscious mind will be alert and attentive to the possibility that you are not playing around. It will begin to bring in support from many places through the law of attraction. Before you know it, you will have what you need to complete your vision. This works for positive things that you desire, and it works for negative things that you don't desire. It all boils down to what your point of focus is. Basically, that is what you will be attracting to yourself.

You must be careful, because you are human. When you change your behaviors, you can achieve success and accomplish great things. If these things are completely foreign to you, you may have a tendency to go back to familiar territory. That familiar territory may not always be the best place for you, though, and could put you back in the same boat you climbed out of. People often relapse after they lose weight because they make changes that they are not able to sustain mentally, physically, and/or spiritually. Truly affirmed changes help us to establish a new comfort zone where we are not recreating old situations that don't serve us effectively.

How to Create Affirmations

There are a few secrets to creating effective affirmations:

1. When you are creating affirmations, you should say them as if they are occurring as you speak. They have already been accomplished. They are as good as done! These affirmations are made in the present tense. "I am healthy, I am well, I am awesome, I am strong, I am woman, etc." The future tense trips your mind up to keep putting your success in the distant future, and you will find yourself always reaching for it but never attaining it. "I will be a good nurse, I will exercise, I will survive, etc." The present is the only space we have to work with. The past has already been created by our thoughts, and the future is being formed by what we are doing now.

2. Affirmations should be positive. The subconscious mind will take negatives and bring those negatives into reality. An example of this would be, "I am not bad at starting IVs." Your mind is actually hearing that you are bad at starting IVs.
3. Say your affirmations daily and often. Write your affirmations down often. (The self-care exercises in the next section will help you fulfill this requirement for effective affirmations.) Listen to your affirmations often. This definitely is a means to program your subconscious mind to receive your affirmation.
4. Gather pictures and create a collage of what you desire or want to achieve. These symbols work as affirmations and are quite effective for your brain. When I first moved into my house, I had nothing in it. I didn't even have blinds for my windows. I got a posterboard and covered it with clippings from magazines and newspapers of everything I wanted in my house. A year later, I pulled the posterboard out of my garage and was amazed to realize that I had everything that I had put on it.
5. Practice makes perfect. Practice creates patterns of familiarity. If you want to learn something really well, continue to do it over and over and over again. You will form a habit. When you first learned how to drive, you had to think about it really hard. Now that you have been driving for years, you probably feel like you could do it in your sleep (as scary as that is to think about). Your subconscious mind knows the routine. Have you ever driven home tired after working a night shift, and realized that you arrived safely but don't really remember driving? I have done that myself before. The subconscious mind is amazing and very protective.
6. Seal your affirmations with a prayer. Speak your affirmations first, and then follow them up with a prayer. Your prayers carry a different tone when you are in a positive state of affirmation. Basically, the prayer gives you a double dose of the "good" stuff. Your vibration will be that much higher, allowing you to create an even clearer channel for fulfillment. This final step was adapted from a book by J. Donald Walters (1988) called *Affirmations for Self-Healing*. Here is how he explains it:

> Why should one pray only after repeating the affirmations? Why not before? Prayer is always good, certainly. But if it isn't uttered with an affirmative consciousness, it can easily become weak and beggarly; a plea that God do all the work, without man's participation. Effective prayer is never passive. It is full of faith. It matures in an attitude of affirmation.

When to Use Affirmations

We use affirmations to bring ourselves up to a higher standard of accomplishment when we have not yet achieved our point of focus. We use them to help us create change inwardly, to improve our relationships with others, to accomplish goals, and to help us fulfill our desires. When we are building ourselves up, we want to take others up with us. Affirmations should be used each and every time you open your mouth to communicate with others. I don't mean that you need to affirm someone to bring you a Diet Coke. I am speaking of the conversations you have that build relationships and build support for you to accomplish the things you desire in your life. There are many instances in which affirmations are important. How many times do you look at someone you are not in harmony with and affirm that the relationship you share is one of peace and bliss? You might be distracted by the negative talk that your mind is feeding you, based on past experience. See what you can do to reshape the future. What we think to ourselves and say to others should always be affirmative, constructive, and compassionate.

Affirmations are used when change is desired or needed. When you want to modify behaviors in yourself or displeasing aspects of your situation for the better, use affirmations as a tool in conjunction with other actions. Affirmations can be extremely useful for improving relationships if you are already doing things to communicate openly, exercise unconditional love, and truly connect with other individuals. Affirmations should never be manipulated for selfish reasons or used against others, because you will experience the law of karma (what you sow you will reap!).

Affirmation Exercises for Self-Care

Thought monitor journal

"Thought is cause" is one of the most important phrases I learned in my studies at the School of Metaphysics. For this exercise, you are going to monitor your thoughts for a day, a week, a month, or however long you desire. Draw a line down the center of a piece of paper and write "Positive" at the top of one side and "Negative" on the other side. Each day, be conscious of the thoughts you are thinking and how they will impact the future that you are creating. For example, if you wake up and subconsciously think, "This day is going to suck!", write that down in the negative column in your journal. If you think to yourself, "Wow, I really learn fast!", write that on the positive side. At the end of the day, write down what impact you think your thoughts might have had on your day or what impact they might have on your future. This will help you become an avid thought watcher. Tally up your thoughts at the end of the day and see how many positive and negative thoughts you have had. The purpose of this exercise is not to make you feel bad but to help you track your progress. You will become more and more aware of your thoughts, which should lead to less negative and more positive ones. This only means that you will attract more of what you want and less of what you don't! Sounds good, doesn't it?

The 100 Affirmations Club

The 100 Affirmations Club is an exercise that lets you sharpen your affirmation writing skills so that you can create a new habit of affirming greatness in your life. Get a pack of 100 (3×5) index cards and write an affirmation on each card. Once you've completed your affirmations, place them in strategic places in your house or your car where you will be sure to see them. People at work may think you're insane. People at home may feel close to committing you, because they don't understand your project. Affirm anyway! I have dedicated a wall in one of my rooms to my affirmations. (If the index card idea doesn't appeal to you, make a list in your journal or on regular notebook paper. Number from 1 to 100 and get to affirming!) You can divide your index cards into different categories and have affirmations for each category in your life you wish to support. These categories could include such things as Finances, Relationships, Education, Health, Spirituality, Career, Recreation, Fitness, and Nutrition. Create affirmations that will support you in areas you need to improve or change. Some example affirmations are given below:

Finances

    My finances improve daily.

    I attract wealth and abundance easily.

    My income meets my needs and more.

Relationships

    My partner and I communicate clearly and with compassion.

    My children and I spend quality time together daily.

    I establish meaningful partnerships with my patients and coworkers.

Education

    I learn quickly and effectively.

    I retain information easily.

    I apply my knowledge appropriately in any situations.

Health

    I am strong and well, inside and out.

    My immune system functions perfectly.

    I do the right things to maintain my health and wellness.

Spirituality

    Meditation is easy and healing.

    I pray every morning with great success.

    My spirit is free from guilt and shame.

Career

My job is satisfying.

I am an awesome nurse.

My value is appreciated by myself and others.

Recreation

I have fun in moderation.

Salsa dancing invigorates and inspires me.

I experience the outdoors daily.

Fitness

I enjoy exercising daily.

I model fitness to my patients by example.

Exercise is convenient and inspiring.

Nutrition

I eat the right foods for my body and blood type.

Sweets and fats are less appealing than veggies and fruits.

Water is refreshing to my body, so I drink adequate amounts.

Speaking is Believing

This exercise requires you to read all of the affirmations you have written on your index cards and record them on a tape/voice recorder or iPod device. Listen to this tape in the morning, at night, or during your breaks at work. Some of you may have the luxury of listening to it all day on a repeat cycle, so that it can soak into your subconscious mind. You don't have to be consciously listening to it all the time, but reciting your affirmations along with your own voice shows a great team effort!

GRATITUDE

> *"Gratitude makes sense of our past, brings peace for today,*
> *and creates a vision for tomorrow."*
>
> — ANONYMOUS

Why Gratitude Is Important

Gratitude is a tool that can help us keep our mood balanced and consistent, and to take a struggling mood and transform it into one that is more positive. Gratitude is also a tool that keeps our channels open and our vibrations up, because we are able to receive from life. We can eliminate the struggles we tend to have when we don't appreciate what we have. Gratitude strengthens our character and helps us to be more positive, because we are focusing on what we have instead of what we don't. Gratitude can serve to buffer the burnout that many nurses experience, which robs them of joy and well-being. In an International Positive Psychology Association newsletter, Lopper (2009) described gratitude as an "orientation towards noticing and appreciating the positive world." We are like tuning forks. When you sound off one tuning fork, the fork next to it begins to resonate at the same pitch. When you exercise gratitude, you resonate at a certain level and can bring everything else around you to that same level.

Just as others can resonate with you, you can resonate at levels that may be less beneficial when you aren't appreciative of what you have. Church is probably one of the main places we learn about gratitude. Every religion or spiritual practice has some lesson or words of wisdom to share relating to gratitude, because it helps us to see the world in a more expansive way. We can better appreciate what we have if we are able to recognize the suffering that other people experience. Home is another place where we learn about gratitude. Remember not wanting to eat all your food, or not wanting to eat meatloaf for the third night in a row? You were destined to get the "gratitude" lecture, in which you were reminded about all the starving people in the world. I remember singing a little song at church called "Count your Blessings." The words went like this:

Count your blessings, name them one by one.
Count your blessings, see what God has done.
Count your blessings, name them one by one.
Count your many blessings, see what God has done.

Every time I wanted to complain, there was always an adult telling me I had so much to be grateful for. That used to really irritate me, because there was no way he or she could tell me that my situation wasn't as bad as I believed it was. Age and time have taught me that what they were trying to explain to me was very true. There is always something to be thankful for, despite whatever turmoil seems to be surrounding you. Magical things happen when you are grateful for what you have. You attract more things to you that are good. You are a clear channel for creativity, for peace, and for an awesome attitude.

Gratitude, as well as any other tool we use, is not a ticket that guarantees we will never experience hardship, discomfort, or sadness. We are human and have these experiences for our soul growth and learning. But by practicing gratitude, we can adjust and recalibrate ourselves so that we can once again return to a place of harmony.

Benefits of Gratitude

Research shows that people can achieve good health by expressing gratitude and thankfulness. According to Lopper (2009), "research is finding a positive relationship between gratitude and a person's cardiovascular and immune functions." There is something to be said about those good vibrations flowing through your body. They can result in an enhanced immune system, improved relationships, creativity, success, mental clarity, and joy.

Gratitude Exercises for Self-Care

Gratitude list

Each day make a list of 10 things for which you are grateful, and why you are grateful for them. At the end of the day, explore the things you noticed during the day and feel the thankfulness that you were able to capture at the time. An example list is provided below:

Ten Things for Which I Am Grateful

1. I am grateful for a healthy back, because I am able to walk, work, and salsa dance with my friends.
2. I am grateful for a supportive manager, because I enjoy work more.
3. I am grateful for my health and strength, because I have no pain and enjoy my life.
4. I am grateful for a reliable vehicle, because I am able to go wherever I want, when I want to.
5. I am grateful for a good career, because it helps me take pride in myself and what I do for others each day.
6. I am grateful for appreciative patients, because I know that I am appreciating myself too.
7. I am grateful for loving children, because I know that they are responding to my love for them.
8. I am grateful my children like to cook and clean, because when I am tired at the end of the day I enjoy coming home to a clean home and good food.
9. I am grateful I passed my board exams the first time, because I was able to get a job immediately and enjoy an increase in my finances.
10. I am grateful I do not have to take the GRE again, because it saved me time and was less stressful.

Spirit sprucin'

Gratitude helps lift our spirits, but sometimes we need a jump start. I have made a list of things you can explore to shift your spirits, which I call "spirit sprucin'." Table 12-1 illustrates things that you can do to spruce up your spirits and place yourself in the flow of appreciation and well-being.

Table 12-1   Spirit Sprucin'

When we wake up on the wrong side of the bed, it can be very tempting to stay on the wrong side for the rest of the day. That day can turn into week, etc. Make a conscious choice to get out of your rut and spruce your spirit. Once you start sprucin', the world begins to turn and the universe recognizes your intentions to make a great day and works with you to honor that. Start sprucin!

1. Set your intention for the day you choose to have.
2. Smile at yourself in the mirror.
3. Sing and dance with yourself in the mirror, restroom, or office.
4. Share an occasional inspirational e-mail with others (that doesn't require them to e-mail 50 people).
5. Listen to music.
6. Wear colors that make you feel good.
7. Go for a quick walk during a break or a long stroll if you are off work.
8. Observe nature and experience the beauty.
9. Take your shoes off and walk on your grass.
10. Hug a tree (yes hug a tree!!)
11. Offer your services to others (serve in a food kitchen, visit a nursing home and share yourself with others, etc).
12. Use a special aromatherapy blend for your home or office.
13. Pass out compliments to others.
14. Notice the good things about people and share with them.
15. Have gratitude for what you have.
16. Get a massage or some other form of self-care.
17. Eat healthy snacks and meals.
18. Hydrate yourself with water.
19. Let someone cut in front of you on the highway.
20. Call someone you haven't spoken to in a long time and say hello.
21. Rearrange your home or your office to change the energy.
22. Breathe deeply and fully, enjoying the breath.
23. Take a bubble bath.
24. Put on smell-goods or perfume!
25. Give smiley face stickers to your coworkers.

"Thank you kindly" exercise

Observe the different things that people do to be supportive of you and make your life easier. Does someone always make sure you get your patients' histories and physicals put away in a nice, neat folder? Does someone call you every time you get a message, so that you don't miss the information you are supposed to receive? Does someone know that you like frogs and manage to give you a little collectible one here and there? These things can often go unnoticed.

All you need to do is give each individual is a simple "Thank you kindly." You may not want to say "thank you kindly" in those exact words, but in your own way say "thank you" to others each day for what they make a point to do for you. It is important to let others know that you recognize and appreciate their supportive efforts.

When I was in college, I had a roommate from Japan. She was very kind and giving, and was always cooking in our room. (I always smelled like whatever she was having for lunch, breakfast, or dinner!) One day I invited her to a potluck gathering with my friends. She couldn't speak English very well, but I knew she wanted to make something for the gathering. She made about a dozen large rice balls wrapped in seaweed paper. My friends tried them, but they weren't very open to this new kind of cuisine. After everyone ate, we put the food away so that it wouldn't go bad and our resident assistant wouldn't come fussing at us. I thanked my roommate for her effort in making the rice balls. Her eyes lit up and she told me she would be right back. In the meantime, we were watching movies in the basement of my dorm. She came back a half hour later with another dozen rice balls! My point is that gratitude attracts people who appreciate that you appreciate them. This gratitude potentiates the effects of more gratitude and spreads across the world.

How many nurses feel disappointment when their work goes unnoticed? So much of what we do goes unnoticed and without praise. Why not praise someone else for what they do, so that you can experience gratitude from a different perspective. Don't forget to say thank you to yourself as well. You have to be grateful for who you are, before you can thoroughly appreciate the goodness of others.

The struggles we experience often come from our inability to accept the things we are unable to change with a willingness and presence to see what we can change. Practicing these four components of spirituality cannot only help us achieve a deeper meaning in our nursing practice, they can also help us move toward a higher consciousness as human beings.

If you are wondering what your existence would be like if you were living at this level of higher consciousness, I would advise you to read a book called *The Four Agreements*, by Don Miguel Ruiz (1997), which presents a clear picture of what spiritual practices can create within an individual. The first of the four agreements is to be impeccable with your word. Don't make promises you can't keep, just because you are afraid to disappoint others and would rather overextend yourself. This also includes refraining from gossiping about others in your family or in the workplace. How much easier would life be if you kept this simple agreement?

The second agreement is to not take everything personally. We tend to blame ourselves when people treat us in unsatisfactory ways, when things don't work out perfectly, or when we can't manage to do it all. Not thinking that everything is about you can definitely benefit your self-esteem.

The third agreement is to not make assumptions. We can get into a cycle of feeling victimized when we expect people to read our minds. Misunderstandings do occur, and often happen when we don't communicate clearly. There are things we can do to prevent or lessen such misunderstandings, though. Say what you mean, as clearly as you can. It helps when you aren't afraid to communicate what you truly want.

The last agreement is to do your best in every situation. This doesn't mean that you should expect to do everything perfectly. Doing your best means that you do what you can at any given time with compassion and presence. You are able to release what you are unable to manage, and to know that things will work out for the best. The spiritual self-care practices of praying, meditating, affirming, and having gratitude create an environment for us in which we can abide by the four agreements as a natural part of our daily lives.

REFERENCES

Anonymous. (2002). Nontraditional choices: practicing meditation. *Nursing, 70*.

Khalsa, H. K. (2006). *A woman's book of meditation: Discover the power of a peaceful mind.* New York: Penguin Group.

Lopper, J. (2009). *Good health: expressing gratitude and thankfulness; how to be healthy with an attitude of appreciation and gratefulness.* Retrieved June 5, 2009, from Suite101. com: http://personaldevelopment.suite101.com/article.cfm/good_health_expressing_gratitude_thankfulness

Ott, M. J. (2004). Mindfulness meditation: a path of transformation and healing. *Journal of Psychosocial Nursing and Mental Health Services, 42*(7), 22–29.

Ruiz, D. M. (1997). *The four agreements.* San Rafael, CA: Amber-Allen.

Tolle, E. (1999). *The power of now.* Novato, CA: New World Library.

Walters, J. D. (1988). *Affirmations for self-healing.* Nevada City, CA: Crystal Clarity.

Wright, S. (2007). Meditation matters. *Nursing Standard,* 18–19.

Practicing What You Preach— Living the Message of Self-Care

RACHEL Y. HILL

"It is no use walking anywhere to preach unless our walking is our preaching."
—ST. FRANCIS OF ASSISI

You have had the opportunity to experience many self-care exercises from your reading. You have the ability to design a "first-aid kit" for emergency situations, when you need to establish balance quickly. You also have tools that will allow you to make long-lasting changes in your personal life and in your career. It's enough to have you as full as a tick (as my grandmother would say)! On a serious note, we have only scratched the surface in establishing the most important relationship you will ever know: the relationship with "me, myself, and I." The rest of this journey is up to you. In the famous words of Smokey the Bear, "Only you can prevent forest fires!" Only you can prevent burnout! I encourage you to take charge of your personal and professional destiny and manifest your true self!

With that being said, I would like to leave you with 10 pearls of wisdom for your journey home. The journey home is, of course, our journey inward. When life seems too complicated and you are in need of an instant regrouping, review the 10 pearls of wisdom and see which one you might need to reconsider and apply to reestablish balance in your life. The pearls I would like to share with you are as follows:

1. Meet YOUR basic needs. It's a new day in the neighborhood. Take care of yourself! Your physical body can only take you so far. Common sense will take you much further if you listen. You can't nurture others if you are running on fumes yourself. Eat a balanced diet (pack a healthy lunch for work). If you find it's easy to pack a healthy lunch for your darling, dimpled children, or your spouse, but somehow you fizzle out when it's time to make yours, commit to making yours first. Drink half your body weight in ounces of water every single day to cleanse your system. Don't forget to use the restroom regularly. We are renouncing "nurse's bladder" forever! Get a good night's rest. Get a catnap in, if you have the luxury. Take your vitamins. Exercise regularly.

2. Have a regularly scheduled leisure/fun, knowing you deserve it. There's nothing like a person who works hard and doesn't know how to let loose and have a good time. There is a short distance between a workaholic and a party pooper. When guiltamortis (guilty feelings that pervade the cells of your being and prevent fun)

273

sets in, it is so easy to lose your perspective. How much can you really accomplish mentally, when you've already worked 12 hours? On those days off when the "Honey Do List" is calling, make sure to schedule in some fun/leisure time for yourself. You can have the best of both worlds! Schedule a massage, take salsa lessons, play beach volleyball, go to a comedy club for the evening.

3. Build your core. The core of your body should be your strongest place. Our will lives in our core. Our diaphragm, gut feelings, and convictions also dwell in this area. If you need to "do the right thing," but find it difficult to do so, you have the will to do it if your core is strong. If there is something you know is not right, you will have the strength to not do it. Appropriate and inappropriate "no's" come from this place. If you are asked to take extra shifts when you've worked three already, you are justified in saying, "No thanks, not this time." Making the choice to nurture yourself at home also requires some core strength. Family and friends expect you to be a nurse on and off the clock. But you are not a machine. Having the strength to make the choices that are right for you, repeatedly, builds your core, just as yogic breathing and stomach crunches build the core. Mirror exercises in which you practice saying "no" can also make you more comfortable with the idea of choosing yourself over others.

4. Practice presence and compassion in all you do. When we are present in our current situations, we don't get stuck in the past or launch ourselves too far into the future. Our patients need us when we are with them. We can't be with them when we are somewhere else. When we are alone with ourselves, we must learn to appreciate the silence. We have an opportunity to look inward and explore what makes us healthy and complete, without looking for a bunch of other tasks to complete just because we can't sit still. Our families need us when we are with them. We can't be with them when we are still at our jobs, with our patients, or preoccupied with other things. When we'd rather be somewhere else but can't be, it is the fault of no one. Acceptance of our current situation can help us to surrender. Sometimes we can have all the patience and compassion in the world for our patients, but have little left for our families. Stop and think. What would Jesus do? What would Buddha do? What would Florence do? When you have your answer, make sure you show yourself the same treatment. Be present and compassionate with yourself.

5. Communicate honestly and openly about your feelings. Speaking to win isn't necessary. Speaking your mind is necessary. Listening is equally important. When you are involved in discussions that are challenging and tense, set your intentions to achieve the highest level of communication possible for everyone involved. Remember that you're not the only one who has convictions; the important thing is to honor the fact that we all have something of great value to say, through the many beautiful means we have

of expressing ourselves. Singing in the rain, singing in the shower, and making angels in the snow still count as creative expression. Do these kinds of activities as often as you can.

6. We don't call it "nurse's intuition" for nothing. As nurses, we have an innate gift to connect with others in the deepest of ways. But sometimes we may not heed, or even understand, our inner voice. The next time that little voice says "go left," go left and see what happens. Don't second-guess yourself and assume you need to go right just because you are always wrong. You just might be surprised. Now if a tiny voice tells you to bake a coworker some brownies, and she or he has been very harsh toward you, take the high road. There has to be a greater purpose in store for you in creating harmony in that relationship. Trusting your inner voice creates an inner rapport that you've been longing to have.

7. My late grandfather always used to say, "Stay away from negative-talking people!" This phrase means exactly what is says. It's best to stay away from negative-talking people, as well as negative, toxic environments. If someone has no trouble running other people down, she or he will have no problem running you down also. Don't participate in the slander of others or the slander of yourself. Be a part of the solution, not the problem. Negativity is a force that can absorb you rather quickly, like a black hole.

8. Thought is cause. Remember that your thoughts are snapshots of the words you will speak to others. The words you speak will paint the portrait of the life you will create and live for yourself. If you speak something that is not in harmony with who you truly are, or you speak something against someone, take a deep breath and be gentle with yourself. Old habits can be broken. Tell yourself you are better than your actions. Make a conscious effort to make a different choice and keep working with yourself on the issue.

9. Connect with the Earth. Mother Nature calls us each time we see a pretty flower or a butterfly flitter across the way. If it seems like you spend all your time going from work to home and then back to work, stopping to smell the roses may seem unrealistic. Make time to connect with the Earth as often and as frequently as possible. When situations seem overwhelming to me, in the workplace or at home, I can go outside and realize that nature's design is perfect. I am also part of nature's design. Go camping to connect with nature, wake up to the birds chirping, and outsmart the mosquitoes. Travel to the ocean, the canyon, or the mountains to absorb the magnificence of the beauty that is available to us. If travel isn't readily an option, get some postcards and visualize your experience. Carry gems or stones from your collection, or even a pouch of herbs that you have grown in your own little herbal pots. Take your shoes off and allow your feet to connect to the Earth. Feel your connection to the Earth's core. Take some of that Mother Nature with you wherever you go!

10. Connect with your spirit and Creator as often as you can. If you don't, you can get caught up in the illusion that you are alone and that we are not connected with one another in this big world. What impacts you impacts me, and impacts the world. Whatever activities keep you connected, do them on a regular basis. If you work a weekend shift and can't make it to church, see if the service can be recorded. If you like to meditate or pray, make good use of the hospital chapel. The spirit is where you are, and that means within.

Take these pearls and wear them on your journey inward. It is my greatest hope that you have read things in this book that resonate with you. I truly have. Each chapter I have written has given me a special message for myself, each and every time I read it. That message is: "Be who you truly are and live through your personal truths!" My second greatest hope is that you will be able to incorporate these self-care practices into your life and begin living life from within. Finally, I hope that you will come to know and experience (if you haven't already) the fact that balance in our world is possible.

"Love yourself—accept yourself—forgive yourself—and be good to yourself, because without you the rest of us are without a source of many wonderful things."
—LEO F. BUSCAGLIA

One day I visited a Web site called Persuasive.net, which promotes a fast way to learn persuasive communication. While exploring the site, I happened to come across a story about Ghandi, as told by Catherine Ingram. I am always inspired by stories about Ghandi, but I was a little skeptical about the truth of the story. I thought it might be one of those "feel good" stories that people send by e-mail asking others to send it to fifty other people or their car won't start in the morning. Nevertheless, it piqued my interest. The title of the story was "Do You Practice What You Preach?" According to the story, a woman went to Ghandi and asked him to tell her son to "please give up eating sugar." Ghandi told her to bring her son back to him in one week. One week later, she returned with her son, and Ghandi asked the boy to "please give up eating sugar." The woman thanked Ghandi and asked him why he hadn't said the same thing the week before. He replied, "Because a week ago, I had not given up eating sugar." That was a very inspiring story, so I investigated a little further. I wanted to share it with others and didn't want to repeat a false story just for the sake of feeling good. I looked up Catherine Ingram who had written the article online and discovered she is the author of *In the Footsteps of Gandhi: Conversations with Spiritual/Social Activists"* and *Passionate Presence: Qualities of Awakened Awareness*. She seems to be a very impressive woman. I felt like she was a credible source. I am so glad the story is true, because it is too inspiring not to share with you.

It is refreshing to witness the integrity that Ghandi displayed with the mother and her child. The message of this story is very profound. Revisit all the times you have scolded your patients for noncompliance, even though you never finished that full course of amoxicillin like you were supposed to. There is an energy that resonates when people share with others what they truly believe in. If you don't believe in a product, it is useless to try to sell it to others. If we don't believe in taking care of ourselves, then our patients are going to third space in their minds or not pay attention to a word we say, when we talk to them about anything. I don't blame them. Why should they heed our warnings about lung cancer when we are lighting up three packs of cigarettes a day? If we are going to practice self-care, we might as well do it right. Practicing self-care the right way means not leaving anyone out, especially ourselves. In fact, if I had my way, I would give nurses the red-carpet, Hollywood star treatment, just to show them how incredibly special they are. We are the divas and gents of health care. It is time we started seeing that in ourselves. Don't get ridiculous and start requesting your own trailer and makeup artist at work. Just know that you are special. When you believe in something strongly enough, you can also convince others that it is a worthwhile venture. Once they experience it for themselves, that convincing becomes conviction and you have a comrade for the cause. So, if you see red carpet on the walkway to your entrance at work, you're gonna know I was there!

SAT NAM

(The truth is our identity.)

Glossary of Terms

Adi mantra – Tuning in before a yoga set or meditation. This mantra is chanted at the beginning of a yoga session to connect us to the divine teacher we have inside. We are able to connect to our yogic lineage through this mantra and tap into the highest guidance, energy, and inspiration. The Adi mantra is "Ong Namo Guru Dev Namo," which means "I call on the infinite creative consciousness."

Alpha state – The state during hypnosis in which we are the most receptive to suggestions. We can be so relaxed that even though we can hear the phone ring, we don't move and stay in our relaxed state.

Asanas – Consciously taken positions that an individual's awareness, emotions, and reflexes.

Aspect – A characteristic, quality, or virtue by which we judge others or ourselves.

Attitudes – Obstructions in the free flow of the life force energy that lead to physical, mental, and emotional imbalances.

Attunement – The process in which the Reiki Master Teacher enters the energy field/aura of his or her students and prepares the chakras in their bodies to receive the universal Reiki energy that will allow them to help bring balance to others.

Aura – An emanation of subtle energy from the body that can be utilized to detect various states of physical, mental, and emotional health.

Autohypnosis – Hypnotizing yourself.

Beta state – A state that describes our waking consciousness. In this state, we go to work, have conversations, plan the menu for dinner, etc.

Bhandas – Contractions of the muscles that direct the flow of psychic energy and change blood circulation, nerve pressure, and cerebral spinal fluid flow.

Biofield – A scientific term for the vibrational emanations that surround and extend beyond the human body, as measured by the superconducting quantum interference device (SQUID) and demonstrated through the mechanism of Kirlian photography.

Blend – A combination of two or more herbs mixed together.

Breath – It is through the breath that the life force is shown forth and expressed.

Burnout – A feeling of emotional exhaustion, depersonalization, and decreased personal accomplishment, sometimes experienced by people who work in occupations that require interaction with other people on a daily basis.

Chakras – Sacred wheels or energy centers of the body that are extensions of the aura, each relating to specific organs and glands of the body, and can be utilized to detect imbalances in the body, mind, and spirit.

Compassion fatigue – Feelings of stress and loss of compassion that affect people in caregiving professions (e.g., nurses, psychotherapists, ministers).

Concentrative meditation – Meditating on a focal point, such as a sound or object, or chanting mantras to develop concentration and awareness.

Conscious mind – The part of your mind that makes decisions on the physical level of consciousness and is capable of self-awareness.

Conversational prayer – Communication with a higher power; such prayers have no structure and cover an array of topics from forgiveness to gratitude.

Decoction – An infusion of simmering roots and/or bark boiling in a menstrum of water for 15–30 minutes to draw the nutrients out to nourish the body.

Delta state – A state of deep sleep.

Depths – The expression of life force energy at different levels of density.

Disease – Disharmony in the body; blocked or stagnated energy.

Dream – A communication from the subconscious mind to the waking mind that occurs during sleep and concerns the conscious state of awareness. This communication is needed to ensure the mental, emotional, and physical well-being of the dreamer.

Ego – The part of your consciousness that wants to control and protect you and the way you have always been.

Electromagnetic field – The force field relating to charges of electricity in motion.

Energy – The life force that flows through the body.

Energy blockage – An interruption or constriction of the natural flow patterns in the human vibrational matrix; may refer to a closed or diminished chakra, asymmetry in the biofield, or nonpolarity and reversal in the meridian flows.

Energy healing – Using energy from an outside source to create a change that promotes harmony and balance within the body.

Energy pathways – The life force energy that goes down the front of the body and up the back, along the 12 organ flows.

Flows – Specific pathways in which the life force energy travels through our bodies.

Gyan Mudra – Meditative hand position in which the tip of the index finger touches the tip of the thumb, resulting in balance and expansion.

Hand positions – There are 16 hand positions in the Usui Reiki system that are used to achieve balance within the body.

Harmony – The state in which the life force energy is able to flow through the body freely.

Herbology – The study of herbs.

Human energy system – The interactive dynamic system of human subtle energies consisting of the chakras, the biofield, and the meridians, which make up the human vibrational matrix of subtle energy.

Hypnosis – The art of getting a person's subconscious mind and conscious mind to work together for a common good and achieve a desired goal.

Hypnotherapist – A licensed professional who is trained to hypnotize others.

Hypnotist – A nonlicensed individual who is trained to hypnotize others.

Infusion – A tea or decoction of herb parts that are boiled for an extended period of time to obtain nutrients from them.

Intention – Holding one's inner awareness and focus to accomplish a specific task or activity; being fully present in the moment.

Intercessory prayer – Communication with a higher power to ask for help for someone else's situation or needs that require change or support.

Jumper cabling – Applying the life force energy throughout the body by means of the hands. One hand is kept grounded on the body while the other moves to different parts. The energy penetrates clothing, casts, shoes, or braces.

Kriya – A set of exercises meant to achieve specific benefits in individuals, practiced within the discipline of yoga.

Kundalini (coiled serpent) – The energy that rests dormant in the root chakra and is released by spiritual exercise and life experience.

Labels – Disharmonies in the body (HIV, cancer, diabetes, etc.); labels can be big or small.

Law of concentrated attention – An idea tends to realize itself when we focus our attention on it.

Law of dominant effect – Accompanying a suggestion with a strong emotion enhances the suggestion. Any prior suggestion is replaced by the combination of the emotion-suggestion.

Law of reverse action – The harder you try to accomplish a task, the more difficult it is to achieve.

Life force – The energy that dwells within all living creatures.

Lineage – The listed (or nonlisted) legacy of attunements that precede students who have become attuned to Reiki (preceded by their teacher).

Mantras – "Man" means mind, and "tra" means to tune the vibration. Mantras are sounds that tune and manage the vibration of the mind, and impact an individual's consciousness.

Meditation – Stilling the mind and concentrating on an object or sound to achieve a state of awareness, self-growth, and higher consciousness.

Meditative prayer – Communion with a higher power; in such prayers, the prayer is quiet and sensitive to the presence of a higher power.

Menstrum – The medium used to extract nutrients from plants.

Meridians – The energy tracts of lines of force by which the life essence travels throughout the entire body; used in acupuncture techniques.

Mindfulness meditation – Meditating by focusing on the breath as a point of concentration.

Mudras – Finger positions that allow us to connect with the body and the mind, impacting the body's energy system.

Non-REM sleep – Stages 1–4 of the sleep cycle, before REM sleep kicks into gear. The stages last about 5–15 minutes.

Nourish – To fortify the body with the nutrients it needs.

Oku Den – Reiki level 2, or second-degree Reiki. This level explores the mental and emotional aspects of self-care, and expands on the physical self-care of oneself and others. Attainment of this level allows one to treat others.

Petitional prayer – Communion with a higher power in relation to a need or concern for spiritual or material help or guidance.

Pranayama – Regulated breathing exercises meant to achieve a purpose within the body.

Prayer – Individual or group communion with a higher power.

Project – A proactive and positive word that allows us to look at issues and situations as solvable. Any issue we face is the work of our lives in progress. Projects are experiences that require planning and objectivity, so that we are able to execute our plans and learn from the project itself. A term that has traditionally been used is "problem." Problems tend to have a negative undertone, with little vibration of hope and victory in overcoming them.

Reiki – Rei is the Christ or Buddha consciousness, and Ki is the universal life force energy.

Reiki principles – Five principles to live by that can help one lead a healthier, more balanced life.

1. Just for today I will accept my many blessings.
2. Just for today I will trust.
3. Just for today I will be at peace.
4. Just for today I will do my work honestly.
5. Just for today I will respect the rights of all life forms.

Reiki symbols – Secret symbols used in Reiki to energize a session, help facilitate mental and emotional healing, and allow the practitioner to help others from a distance.

REM sleep – The stage of sleep in which dreams occur.

Ritual prayer – Communion with a higher power; such prayers are memorized and recited by individuals or groups.

Sadhana – Spiritual exercises that are practiced daily, usually in the early morning, and include yoga, meditation, mantras, and other spiritual practices.

Safety energy locks – The body has 26 special places, identical on each side of the body, that are used to protect the body when it is in disharmony. They are often compared with circuit breakers. When there is a surge, the circuit switches off to protect the source. When energy is blocked in the body, the safety energy lock produces a symptom that alerts us to the disharmony.

Self-care deprivation – The failure to meet one's self-care needs, due to lack of education or physical/mental/emotional/spiritual constraints.

Sensei – Japanese title that is used to address teachers, professors, and other professionals, such as doctors and attorneys.

Shinpiden – Reiki level 3, or Master levels, meaning mystery teaching. This level accommodates the exploration and healing of others and oneself on spiritual, physical, mental, and emotional levels. The Master level and Master Teacher level are both included in this category.

Shoden – Reiki level 1, or first-degree Reiki, used primarily for self-care practices to promote and explore the potential for self-healing.

Stillness – A state of quietness from mental chatter that allows an individual to hear his or her inner guidance.

Stress – Mental, emotional, and physical stimuli that pose a threat to an individual.

Subconscious mind – The part of the mind that maintains bodily functions when we sleep, and goes out and about when we are dreaming; its purpose is to permanently store understandings gleaned from conscious experiences.

Subtle energy – Faint electromagnetic energy fields that exist within living creatures.

Tea – An infusion of flowers and/or leaves boiled in a menstrum of water for 10–15 minutes to draw the nutrients out to drink and for relaxation.

Theta state – A slower state than the alpha state; in this state, we do things automatically but not consciously (for example, forgetting what we just did within the last 3 minutes, driving and not remembering the ride home).

Tincture – An infusion of herbs extracted in a menstrum of alcohol to draw the nutrients out.

Tonic – Substance made from herbs to tone the body.

Trance – A state of altered consciousness in which an individual is relaxed and not totally connected to his or her physical surroundings.

Universal life force energy – The energy that is active within every living being.

Index